CONTENTS

Chapter 1: Introduction to Cluster Headaches   1
Chapter 2: Anatomy and Physiology of Cluster Headaches   10
Chapter 3: Pathophysiology of Cluster Headaches   26
Chapter 4: Clinical Presentation and Diagnosis   44
Chapter 5: Acute and Preventive Treatment Approaches   57
Chapter 6: Lifestyle Modifications and Holistic Management   74
Chapter 7: Comorbidities and Psychosocial Impact   89
Chapter 8: Future Directions and Research Perspectives   102

CHAPTER 1: INTRODUCTION TO CLUSTER HEADACHES

Definition and Classification

Cluster headaches are a debilitating form of primary headache disorder characterized by recurrent, severe, unilateral pain typically located around the eye or temple. Understanding the precise definition and classification of cluster headaches is essential for accurate diagnosis and effective management.

Definition:

Cluster headaches are often referred to as "suicide headaches" due to their intense pain, which is frequently described as excruciating and debilitating. The term "cluster" refers to the characteristic pattern of attacks, wherein multiple headaches occur in clusters or bouts lasting for weeks to months, separated by periods of remission.

The defining features of cluster headaches include:

1. **Unilateral Pain:** The pain associated with cluster headaches is usually unilateral, meaning it affects only one side of the head. It often centers around the eye, temple, or forehead.
2. **Severe Intensity:** Cluster headaches are among the most severe types of headaches. Patients often describe the pain

as piercing, stabbing, or burning in nature, and it can reach maximum intensity within minutes.
3. **Short Duration:** Unlike migraines, which can last for hours to days, cluster headache attacks typically have a shorter duration, ranging from 15 minutes to three hours. However, the frequency of attacks during a cluster period can vary greatly.
4. **Autonomic Symptoms:** Cluster headaches are associated with autonomic symptoms such as lacrimation (tearing), nasal congestion, rhinorrhea (runny nose), ptosis (drooping eyelid), and miosis (constriction of the pupil) on the affected side.
5. **Circadian Rhythm:** Cluster headaches often follow a circadian rhythm, with attacks commonly occurring at specific times of day or night, often waking patients from sleep.

Classification:

Classifying cluster headaches is essential for both clinical diagnosis and research purposes. The International Classification of Headache Disorders (ICHD) provides standardized criteria for the diagnosis of various headache disorders, including cluster headaches. According to the ICHD-3 criteria, cluster headaches are classified as follows:

1. **Episodic Cluster Headaches:** This subtype accounts for the majority of cluster headache cases. Episodic cluster headaches are characterized by periods of frequent attacks (cluster periods) followed by remission periods lasting weeks to months. The duration and frequency of cluster periods can vary between individuals.
2. **Chronic Cluster Headaches:** In contrast to episodic cluster headaches, chronic cluster headaches involve attacks that occur continuously without remission periods or with remission periods lasting less than three months over a

year.
3. **Probable Cluster Headaches:** Some patients may experience cluster-like headache attacks that do not fully meet the criteria for a definitive diagnosis of cluster headaches. These cases are classified as "probable cluster headaches" and may require further evaluation.

Clinical Relevance:

Accurate diagnosis and classification of cluster headaches are crucial for guiding treatment decisions and optimizing patient care. Differentiating cluster headaches from other primary headache disorders, such as migraines or trigeminal neuralgia, is essential to ensure appropriate management strategies are employed.

Furthermore, understanding the episodic or chronic nature of cluster headaches can influence treatment approaches. While acute therapies may be sufficient for managing episodic cluster headaches during active cluster periods, chronic cluster headaches often require more aggressive preventive treatments to alleviate symptoms and improve quality of life.

In summary, defining and classifying cluster headaches according to their clinical characteristics and patterns of occurrence is fundamental for accurate diagnosis, treatment selection, and prognosis determination. By adhering to standardized criteria and guidelines, healthcare professionals can effectively manage cluster headaches and provide optimal care for affected individuals.

Epidemiology and Prevalence

Understanding the epidemiology and prevalence of cluster headaches is crucial for assessing the burden of this condition on affected individuals and healthcare systems, identifying risk factors, and guiding public health initiatives aimed at improving diagnosis and management.

Epidemiology:

Cluster headaches are relatively rare compared to other primary headache disorders, such as migraines and tension-type headaches. However, they are recognized as one of the most severe and disabling types of headache, significantly impacting the quality of life of affected individuals.

Prevalence:

The prevalence of cluster headaches varies geographically and demographically, with some populations exhibiting higher rates than others. Studies have reported prevalence rates ranging from 0.1% to 0.3% in the general population, making cluster headaches relatively uncommon compared to migraines, which affect approximately 12% of adults worldwide.

Demographic Patterns:

Cluster headaches have been observed to occur more frequently in certain demographic groups, including:

1. **Gender:** Historically, cluster headaches were believed to predominantly affect males, with a male-to-female ratio of approximately 3:1. However, more recent studies suggest that the gender distribution may be more balanced, particularly among patients with chronic cluster headaches.
2. **Age:** Cluster headaches can occur at any age, but they typically manifest in adults between the ages of 20 and 50 years. Rare cases of pediatric cluster headaches have also been reported, although they are less common.
3. **Family History:** There is evidence to suggest a genetic predisposition to cluster headaches, as a family

history of the condition is relatively common among affected individuals. However, the precise genetic factors contributing to cluster headaches remain incompletely understood.

Geographical Variation:

The prevalence of cluster headaches exhibits geographical variation, with higher rates reported in certain regions of the world. For example, studies have identified a higher prevalence of cluster headaches in northern European countries, such as Sweden and Norway, compared to other regions.

Risk Factors:

Several factors have been identified as potential risk factors for the development of cluster headaches, including:

1. **Smoking:** Cigarette smoking has been strongly associated with an increased risk of cluster headaches. Smokers are more likely to develop cluster headaches and tend to experience more severe and refractory symptoms compared to non-smokers.
2. **Alcohol Consumption:** Alcohol consumption, particularly during active cluster periods, is a well-known trigger for cluster headache attacks. Certain types of alcoholic beverages, such as red wine and beer, have been reported to be particularly provocative.
3. **Occupational Exposure:** Some occupational exposures, such as working in environments with high levels of airborne irritants or pollutants, have been implicated as potential triggers for cluster headaches. However, further research is needed to elucidate the specific mechanisms underlying these associations.

Impact on Quality of Life:

Cluster headaches impose a significant burden on affected

individuals, impacting various aspects of their daily lives, including:

1. **Physical Functioning:** The intense pain and associated symptoms of cluster headaches can severely limit an individual's ability to engage in daily activities, work, and social interactions.
2. **Emotional Well-being:** The unpredictable nature of cluster headache attacks and their debilitating effects can lead to feelings of frustration, anxiety, and depression among affected individuals.
3. **Social Functioning:** The episodic nature of cluster headaches, coupled with their severity, can disrupt social relationships and activities, leading to social isolation and withdrawal.
4. **Economic Costs:** The economic burden of cluster headaches is substantial, encompassing direct healthcare costs, such as medical consultations, diagnostic tests, and treatments, as well as indirect costs related to productivity losses and absenteeism from work.

Conclusion:

Epidemiological studies have provided valuable insights into the prevalence, demographic patterns, risk factors, and impact of cluster headaches on affected individuals and society. By understanding these epidemiological characteristics, healthcare professionals can better identify and support individuals with cluster headaches, advocate for improved access to care, and develop targeted interventions aimed at reducing the burden of this debilitating condition.

Impact on Quality of Life

Cluster headaches exert a profound impact on the quality of life of affected individuals, encompassing physical, emotional, social, and economic dimensions. Understanding the multifaceted consequences of this debilitating condition is essential for providing comprehensive care and support to those living with cluster headaches.

Physical Impairment:

The hallmark of cluster headaches is excruciating pain, often described as burning, stabbing, or drilling, typically localized around the eye, temple, or forehead. These intense headaches can last from 15 minutes to three hours and may occur multiple times a day during active cluster periods. The severity and frequency of attacks can incapacitate individuals, rendering them unable to carry out routine activities of daily living. The relentless nature of cluster headaches can lead to physical exhaustion and debilitation, further exacerbating the burden on affected individuals.

Emotional Distress:

Living with cluster headaches can evoke a range of negative emotions, including frustration, despair, and hopelessness. The unpredictability and intensity of attacks can instill fear and anxiety in individuals, anticipating the next excruciating episode. Chronic pain and disability associated with cluster headaches can erode self-esteem and self-efficacy, leading to feelings of helplessness and depression. Moreover, the emotional toll of cluster headaches extends beyond the individuals experiencing the condition, impacting their loved ones who witness their suffering and may feel powerless to alleviate it.

Social Isolation:

The episodic nature of cluster headaches, coupled with their debilitating effects, can disrupt social relationships and activities, leading to social isolation and withdrawal. Individuals with cluster headaches may hesitate to engage in social gatherings or commitments, fearing the onset of an attack in public settings. The need for rest and solitude during cluster periods may strain interpersonal relationships, as friends and family struggle to understand the severity and unpredictability of the condition. Consequently, social support networks may diminish, exacerbating feelings of loneliness and alienation among affected individuals.

Occupational Impairment:

Cluster headaches can significantly impact occupational functioning, jeopardizing employment stability and career advancement. The frequency and severity of attacks may necessitate frequent absenteeism from work, leading to productivity losses and financial strain. Moreover, individuals with cluster headaches may struggle to maintain concentration and focus during active cluster periods, impairing their performance and efficiency on the job. The reluctance to disclose the nature of their condition to employers or colleagues due to stigma or fear of discrimination may further exacerbate workplace challenges.

Financial Burden:

The economic burden of cluster headaches extends beyond direct healthcare costs to encompass indirect costs associated with productivity losses and absenteeism from work. Individuals with cluster headaches may incur expenses related to medical consultations, diagnostic tests, prescription medications, and alternative therapies. Furthermore, the financial impact of reduced earning capacity and disability benefits may exacerbate financial insecurity and strain household finances. The cumulative effect of these financial stressors can perpetuate a cycle of socioeconomic disadvantage and exacerbate disparities in access to care.

Coping Strategies:

Despite the profound impact of cluster headaches on quality of life, individuals develop various coping strategies to manage their symptoms and mitigate their adverse effects. These may include:

1. **Medication Management:** Utilizing acute and preventive medications to alleviate pain and reduce the frequency and severity of attacks.
2. **Lifestyle Modifications:** Adopting healthy lifestyle habits, such as regular sleep patterns, stress management techniques, and dietary adjustments, to minimize trigger factors and enhance overall well-being.
3. **Support Networks:** Seeking support from healthcare providers, support groups, and online communities to connect with others experiencing similar challenges and share coping strategies and emotional support.
4. **Psychological Interventions:** Engaging in psychotherapy, counseling, or relaxation techniques to address underlying emotional distress and develop resilience in coping with cluster headaches.

Conclusion:

Cluster headaches exert a significant and multifaceted impact on the quality of life of affected individuals, encompassing physical, emotional, social, and economic dimensions. Recognizing the complex interplay between these domains is essential for providing holistic care and support to those living with cluster headaches. By addressing the diverse needs of affected individuals and fostering a supportive environment, healthcare providers can empower individuals to manage their condition effectively and enhance their overall quality of life.

CHAPTER 2: ANATOMY AND PHYSIOLOGY OF CLUSTER HEADACHES

Overview of Cranial Anatomy

Understanding the cranial anatomy is fundamental for comprehending the pathophysiology of cluster headaches, as well as for accurate diagnosis and effective management of this condition. This subchapter provides a comprehensive overview of the anatomical structures relevant to cluster headaches, highlighting their roles in pain perception and modulation.

Skull:

The skull serves as the protective framework for the brain and surrounding structures. It is composed of several bones, including the frontal, parietal, temporal, and occipital bones, as well as the sphenoid and ethmoid bones. The cranial vault encloses the brain, while the cranial base forms the floor of the skull and contains various foramina through which cranial nerves and blood vessels pass.

Brain:

The brain is the central organ of the nervous system and is

responsible for processing sensory information, initiating motor responses, and regulating vital functions. It is divided into several major regions, including the cerebrum, cerebellum, and brainstem. The cerebrum, which comprises the largest portion of the brain, is further divided into lobes, including the frontal, parietal, temporal, and occipital lobes, each with distinct functions related to cognition, sensation, and motor control.

Cranial Nerves:

Twelve pairs of cranial nerves emerge from the brainstem and supply sensory and motor innervation to the head and neck. Several cranial nerves play a crucial role in the pathophysiology of cluster headaches, including:

1. **Trigeminal Nerve (CN V):** The trigeminal nerve is the largest cranial nerve and is responsible for transmitting sensory information from the face to the brain. It consists of three divisions: the ophthalmic (V1), maxillary (V2), and mandibular (V3) divisions. The trigeminal nerve plays a central role in the generation and transmission of pain signals in cluster headaches.
2. **Facial Nerve (CN VII):** The facial nerve innervates the muscles of facial expression and plays a role in lacrimation (tearing) and nasal congestion, common autonomic symptoms of cluster headaches.
3. **Oculomotor Nerve (CN III), Trochlear Nerve (CN IV), and Abducens Nerve (CN VI):** These cranial nerves control the movements of the eyes and are implicated in the ocular manifestations of cluster headaches, such as ptosis (drooping eyelid) and ophthalmoplegia (paralysis of eye muscles).

Blood Supply:

The brain receives a rich blood supply from the internal carotid arteries and vertebral arteries, which give rise to the anterior and posterior circulation, respectively. The Circle of Willis, a network of interconnected arteries at the base of the brain, provides redundancy in blood flow and ensures adequate perfusion to critical areas of the brain. Disruption of blood flow or vascular abnormalities in the cranial circulation may contribute to the pathogenesis of cluster headaches.

Trigeminal Autonomic Reflex Pathway:

The trigeminal autonomic reflex pathway (TARP) is a neural circuit implicated in the generation of autonomic symptoms characteristic of cluster headaches. It involves the trigeminal nerve (CN V) and autonomic fibers from the superior cervical ganglion, which converge in the trigeminal ganglion and project to the ipsilateral hypothalamus. Activation of this pathway leads to the release of neuropeptides and neurotransmitters involved in pain transmission and autonomic regulation, contributing to the clinical manifestations of cluster headaches.

Anatomical Variations and Implications:

Individuals may exhibit variations in cranial anatomy, such as variations in the course or branching patterns of cranial nerves, skull anomalies, or vascular malformations. These anatomical variations may influence the presentation, severity, or response to treatment in patients with cluster headaches. Moreover, knowledge of anatomical landmarks is essential for accurate localization of pain and targeted interventions, such as nerve blocks or surgical procedures.

Conclusion:

A thorough understanding of cranial anatomy is essential for elucidating the pathophysiology of cluster headaches and guiding clinical management. The intricate network of cranial structures, including the brain, cranial nerves, and blood vessels, plays a pivotal role in the generation and transmission of pain signals associated with cluster headaches. By integrating anatomical knowledge with clinical assessment, healthcare providers can optimize diagnostic accuracy and therapeutic efficacy in the management of this debilitating condition.

Neurovascular Anatomy of the Head and Neck

The neurovascular anatomy of the head and neck encompasses a complex network of blood vessels and neural structures that play a critical role in the pathophysiology of cluster headaches. This subchapter provides a comprehensive overview of the neurovascular anatomy relevant to cluster headaches, highlighting the interactions between nerves and blood vessels that contribute to the initiation and propagation of pain signals.

Arterial Supply:

The arterial supply to the head and neck originates from the common carotid arteries and vertebral arteries, which give rise to the internal and external carotid arteries. These arteries supply oxygenated blood to the brain, face, and surrounding structures, including the meninges and cranial nerves.

Internal Carotid Artery:

The internal carotid artery gives rise to several branches that supply blood to the brain and orbit. The ophthalmic artery, a branch of the internal carotid artery, provides blood to the orbit, including the structures surrounding the eye. Disruption of blood flow in the ophthalmic artery or its branches may contribute to the ocular symptoms experienced by individuals with cluster headaches.

External Carotid Artery:

The external carotid artery supplies blood to the face, scalp, and superficial structures of the head and neck. Its branches include the superficial temporal artery, which supplies blood to the scalp, and the maxillary artery, which provides blood to the deep structures of the face, including the maxillary sinus and teeth. Dysfunction or dilation of these arteries may contribute to the facial pain and autonomic symptoms characteristic of cluster headaches.

Venous Drainage:

Venous drainage from the head and neck is facilitated by a network of veins that converge into the internal jugular vein. These veins drain deoxygenated blood from the brain, face, and scalp and play a role in regulating intracranial pressure and cerebral perfusion. Dysfunction of venous drainage may contribute to intracranial hypertension, a potential trigger for cluster headache attacks.

Trigeminal Nerve (CN V):

The trigeminal nerve is the largest cranial nerve and plays a central role in the pathophysiology of cluster headaches. It is divided into three divisions: the ophthalmic (V1), maxillary (V2), and mandibular (V3) divisions. The ophthalmic division supplies sensory innervation to the forehead, scalp, and orbit, while the maxillary and mandibular divisions supply sensation to the face and oral cavity. Dysfunction or sensitization of the trigeminal nerve may lead to the generation and transmission of pain signals characteristic of cluster headaches.

Autonomic Nervous System:

The autonomic nervous system regulates involuntary functions, including blood vessel tone, heart rate, and respiratory rate. Dysregulation of the autonomic nervous system is implicated in the autonomic symptoms associated with cluster headaches, such as lacrimation, nasal congestion, and ptosis. The trigeminal-autonomic reflex pathway, which involves connections between the trigeminal nerve and autonomic nuclei in the brainstem and hypothalamus, plays a key role in mediating these autonomic responses.

Cervical Sympathetic Chain:

The cervical sympathetic chain consists of a series of ganglia located along the length of the vertebral column. It plays a role in regulating blood vessel tone and pupil dilation, functions that are dysregulated in individuals with cluster headaches. Dysfunction of the cervical sympathetic chain may contribute to the autonomic symptoms experienced during cluster headache attacks.

Vascular Innervation:

Blood vessels in the head and neck are innervated by sensory and autonomic nerves that regulate vascular tone and blood flow. Sensory fibers from the trigeminal nerve and autonomic fibers from the sympathetic and parasympathetic nervous systems converge on blood vessels, modulating their diameter and reactivity. Dysfunction of vascular innervation may lead to vasodilation, inflammation, and neurogenic inflammation, processes implicated in the pathogenesis of cluster headaches.

Conclusion:

The neurovascular anatomy of the head and neck is intricately linked to the pathophysiology of cluster headaches, with interactions between nerves and blood vessels playing a central role in pain generation and transmission. A thorough understanding of this anatomy is essential for elucidating the mechanisms underlying cluster headaches and guiding targeted therapeutic interventions aimed at alleviating symptoms and improving patient outcomes. By integrating knowledge of neurovascular anatomy with clinical assessment, healthcare providers can optimize diagnostic accuracy and therapeutic efficacy in the management of this debilitating condition.

Trigeminal Autonomic Reflex Pathway

The trigeminal autonomic reflex pathway (TARP) is a neural circuit implicated in the generation and modulation of autonomic symptoms associated with cluster headaches. Understanding the intricate connections and neurotransmitter signaling within this pathway is crucial for unraveling the pathophysiology of cluster headaches and developing targeted therapeutic interventions. This subchapter provides a comprehensive overview of the trigeminal autonomic reflex pathway, highlighting its role in pain transmission, autonomic regulation, and the pathogenesis of cluster headaches.

Anatomy of the Trigeminal Nerve:

The trigeminal nerve (CN V) is the fifth cranial nerve and is responsible for transmitting sensory information from the face to the brain. It is divided into three main branches: the ophthalmic nerve (V1), the maxillary nerve (V2), and the mandibular nerve (V3). These branches innervate different regions of the face and oral cavity, conveying sensory signals related to touch, temperature, and pain.

Trigeminal Ganglion:

The cell bodies of sensory neurons of the trigeminal nerve are located in the trigeminal ganglion, which is situated within the middle cranial fossa. The trigeminal ganglion serves as a relay station for sensory input from the face and sends projections to various regions of the brainstem, including the spinal trigeminal nucleus and the trigeminal nucleus caudalis.

Autonomic Nuclei:

The trigeminal autonomic reflex pathway involves connections between the trigeminal nerve and autonomic nuclei located within the brainstem and hypothalamus. These nuclei include the superior salivatory nucleus, the dorsal raphe nucleus, and the paraventricular nucleus of the hypothalamus. These nuclei integrate sensory input from the trigeminal nerve with autonomic signals and modulate autonomic responses, such as lacrimation, nasal congestion, and pupillary changes.

Neurotransmitter Signaling:

Neurotransmitters play a key role in mediating the transmission of signals within the trigeminal autonomic reflex pathway. Glutamate is the primary excitatory neurotransmitter involved in transmitting sensory signals from the trigeminal nerve to the brainstem. Substance P and calcitonin gene-related peptide (CGRP) are neuropeptides released from trigeminal sensory neurons and contribute to neurogenic inflammation and pain sensitization. Serotonin (5-HT) is another neurotransmitter implicated in modulating pain perception and autonomic function within the brainstem.

Activation of the Trigeminal Autonomic Reflex Pathway:

The trigeminal autonomic reflex pathway can be activated by various stimuli, including noxious stimuli, environmental triggers, and changes in circadian rhythm. Activation of sensory neurons within the trigeminal ganglion leads to the release of neurotransmitters and neuropeptides, which propagate signals along the trigeminal nerve fibers to the brainstem and hypothalamus. Efferent pathways originating from autonomic nuclei result in the manifestation of autonomic symptoms, such as lacrimation, nasal congestion, and ptosis.

Role in Cluster Headaches:

The trigeminal autonomic reflex pathway is believed to play a central role in the pathogenesis of cluster headaches. Activation of this pathway leads to the release of vasoactive peptides, such as CGRP, causing vasodilation and neurogenic inflammation in the cranial vasculature. Additionally, the release of neurotransmitters, such as glutamate and substance P, sensitizes trigeminal nociceptive pathways, leading to the perception of pain. Dysregulation or hyperactivity of the trigeminal autonomic reflex pathway may contribute to the development and exacerbation of cluster headaches.

Therapeutic Implications:

Targeting the trigeminal autonomic reflex pathway represents a promising therapeutic strategy for the management of cluster headaches. Pharmacological agents that modulate neurotransmitter release or receptor activity within this pathway, such as CGRP antagonists or serotonin agonists, have shown efficacy in reducing the frequency and severity of cluster headache attacks. Additionally, neuromodulation techniques, such as occipital nerve stimulation or deep brain stimulation, may modulate activity within the trigeminal autonomic reflex pathway and alleviate symptoms in refractory cases.

Conclusion:

The trigeminal autonomic reflex pathway is a complex neural circuit implicated in the pathogenesis of cluster headaches. Understanding the anatomical connections, neurotransmitter signaling, and activation mechanisms within this pathway is crucial for developing targeted therapeutic interventions aimed at alleviating pain and autonomic symptoms associated with cluster headaches. By elucidating the role of the trigeminal autonomic reflex pathway in cluster headache pathophysiology, researchers and clinicians can advance our understanding of this debilitating condition and improve treatment outcomes for affected individuals.

Role of Hypothalamus and Circadian Rhythm Regulation

The hypothalamus is a small but critically important region of the brain responsible for regulating various physiological processes, including sleep-wake cycles, hormone production, and autonomic function. In the context of cluster headaches, the hypothalamus plays a pivotal role in modulating circadian rhythms and may contribute to the timing and frequency of headache attacks. This subchapter explores the intricate relationship between the hypothalamus, circadian rhythm regulation, and cluster headaches, shedding light on potential mechanisms underlying the circadian pattern of this debilitating condition.

Anatomy of the Hypothalamus:

The hypothalamus is located beneath the thalamus and forms part of the diencephalon. It consists of several nuclei that regulate diverse functions, including the suprachiasmatic nucleus (SCN), which serves as the master circadian pacemaker, and the paraventricular nucleus (PVN), which integrates autonomic and neuroendocrine responses. The hypothalamus receives input from various sensory modalities, including light input from the retina via the retinohypothalamic tract, enabling it to synchronize circadian rhythms with environmental cues.

Circadian Rhythms:

Circadian rhythms are endogenous biological rhythms that oscillate with a periodicity of approximately 24 hours, regulating physiological and behavioral processes in synchrony with the day-night cycle. The suprachiasmatic nucleus (SCN) of the hypothalamus plays a central role in coordinating circadian rhythms by generating rhythmic output signals that influence peripheral clocks throughout the body. These rhythms are entrained by external cues, such as light exposure, which serves as the primary synchronizer or zeitgeber for the circadian system.

Hypothalamic Involvement in Cluster Headaches:

The hypothalamus has long been implicated in the pathophysiology of cluster headaches, given its role in regulating autonomic function and circadian rhythms. Several lines of evidence suggest a close association between hypothalamic dysfunction and cluster headache attacks:

1. **Circadian Pattern:** Cluster headaches often exhibit a distinct circadian pattern, with attacks frequently occurring at specific times of day or night, typically during the rapid eye movement (REM) phase of sleep or shortly after waking. This temporal clustering of attacks suggests involvement of the hypothalamus in modulating the timing and frequency of headache episodes.
2. **Autonomic Symptoms:** The hypothalamus plays a key role in regulating autonomic function, and autonomic symptoms such as lacrimation, nasal congestion, and ptosis are common features of cluster headaches. Dysfunction of hypothalamic nuclei involved in autonomic regulation may contribute to the expression of these symptoms during headache attacks.
3. **Neuroendocrine Alterations:** Cluster headaches have been associated with alterations in neuroendocrine function, including changes in cortisol levels and melatonin secretion, both of which are regulated by the hypothalamus. Dysregulation of the hypothalamic-pituitary-adrenal (HPA) axis and the pineal gland may influence the susceptibility to cluster headache attacks and contribute to their circadian pattern.

Neurotransmitter Systems:

The hypothalamus contains numerous neurotransmitter systems

that modulate circadian rhythms and pain processing, including serotonin, dopamine, and neuropeptides such as orexin and hypocretin. Dysregulation of these neurotransmitter systems may disrupt circadian rhythms and contribute to the development of cluster headaches.

Potential Mechanisms:

Several mechanisms have been proposed to explain the role of the hypothalamus in cluster headaches:

1. **Hypothalamic Activation:** Imaging studies have demonstrated increased hypothalamic activation during cluster headache attacks, suggesting a direct involvement of the hypothalamus in the generation or modulation of pain signals.
2. **Trigeminal Autonomic Reflex Pathway:** The hypothalamus receives input from trigeminal sensory neurons and projects efferent signals to autonomic nuclei involved in cluster headache pathogenesis. Dysfunction of this pathway may contribute to the autonomic symptoms and circadian pattern of cluster headaches.
3. **Neuroendocrine Dysregulation:** Alterations in neuroendocrine function, such as changes in cortisol and melatonin levels, may disrupt circadian rhythms and contribute to the timing and frequency of cluster headache attacks.

Therapeutic Implications:

Targeting the hypothalamus and its associated pathways may represent a promising therapeutic strategy for the management of cluster headaches. Neuromodulation techniques, such as deep brain stimulation or transcranial magnetic stimulation, have been investigated as potential treatments for refractory cluster headaches by modulating hypothalamic activity. Additionally, pharmacological agents that target neurotransmitter systems involved in circadian rhythm regulation and pain processing may offer therapeutic benefit in the management of cluster headaches.

Conclusion:

The hypothalamus plays a central role in regulating circadian rhythms and autonomic function and is implicated in the pathophysiology of cluster headaches. Dysregulation of hypothalamic function may contribute to the circadian pattern, autonomic symptoms, and neuroendocrine alterations observed in cluster headache patients. Further research into the underlying mechanisms of hypothalamic involvement in cluster headaches may lead to the development of novel therapeutic interventions aimed at improving the management and outcomes of this debilitating condition.

Neurotransmitters and Neuromodulators Involved

Neurotransmitters and neuromodulators play a crucial role in the pathophysiology of cluster headaches by mediating pain transmission, modulating neuronal excitability, and regulating autonomic function. Understanding the intricate interplay between these signaling molecules is essential for unraveling the mechanisms underlying cluster headaches and developing targeted therapeutic interventions. This subchapter provides an in-depth exploration of the neurotransmitters and neuromodulators implicated in cluster headaches, shedding light on their roles and potential therapeutic implications.

Serotonin (5-HT):

Serotonin, also known as 5-hydroxytryptamine (5-HT), is a neurotransmitter involved in regulating mood, sleep-wake cycles, and pain processing. Dysregulation of the serotonergic system has been implicated in the pathogenesis of cluster headaches, with alterations in serotonin levels observed during headache attacks. Serotonin receptors, particularly the 5-HT1B/1D receptors, are targets for triptans, a class of medications commonly used to abort cluster headache attacks by constricting cranial blood vessels and inhibiting nociceptive neurotransmission.

Dopamine:

Dopamine is a neurotransmitter involved in reward processing, motor control, and mood regulation. Dysregulation of the dopaminergic system has been implicated in cluster headaches, with alterations in dopamine levels observed during headache attacks. Dopamine receptors, particularly the D2 receptors, are targets for medications such as dopamine antagonists and ergot derivatives, which modulate dopaminergic signaling and may alleviate cluster headache symptoms by inhibiting pain transmission and vasodilation.

Glutamate:

Glutamate is the primary excitatory neurotransmitter in the central nervous system and plays a key role in synaptic transmission and neuronal excitability. Dysregulation of glutamatergic signaling has been implicated in the pathophysiology of cluster headaches, with alterations in glutamate levels observed in animal models and human studies. Glutamate receptors, particularly the N-methyl-D-aspartate (NMDA) receptors, are potential targets for novel therapeutics aimed at modulating pain processing and central sensitization in cluster headaches.

Calcitonin Gene-Related Peptide (CGRP):

Calcitonin gene-related peptide (CGRP) is a neuropeptide involved in vasodilation, neurogenic inflammation, and pain transmission. Elevated levels of CGRP have been implicated in the pathogenesis of cluster headaches, with increased CGRP release observed during headache attacks. CGRP receptor antagonists, such as gepants, represent a novel class of medications that block CGRP signaling and have shown efficacy in aborting cluster headache attacks and preventing their recurrence.

Substance P:

Substance P is a neuropeptide involved in nociception, neurogenic inflammation, and modulation of pain transmission. Dysregulation of substance P signaling has been implicated in the pathophysiology of cluster headaches, with elevated levels of substance P observed in the trigeminal system during headache attacks. Substance P receptor antagonists, such as tachykinin receptor antagonists, may offer therapeutic benefit in cluster headaches by blocking substance P-mediated pain transmission and neurogenic inflammation.

Orexin/Hypocretin:

Orexin, also known as hypocretin, is a neuropeptide involved in regulating wakefulness, arousal, and appetite. Dysregulation of the orexinergic system has been implicated in cluster headaches, with alterations in orexin levels observed during headache attacks. Orexin receptor antagonists, such as suvorexant, may modulate sleep-wake cycles and offer therapeutic benefit in cluster headaches by stabilizing circadian rhythms and reducing the frequency of nocturnal attacks.

GABA (Gamma-Aminobutyric Acid):

GABA is the primary inhibitory neurotransmitter in the central nervous system and plays a key role in modulating neuronal excitability and synaptic transmission. Dysregulation of GABAergic signaling has been implicated in the pathophysiology of cluster headaches, with alterations in GABA levels observed in animal models and human studies. GABA receptor agonists, such as benzodiazepines and gabapentinoids, may offer therapeutic benefit in cluster headaches by enhancing GABAergic inhibition and reducing neuronal hyperexcitability.

Endocannabinoids:

Endocannabinoids are lipid signaling molecules that modulate pain perception, inflammation, and mood regulation. Dysregulation of the endocannabinoid system has been implicated in cluster headaches, with alterations in endocannabinoid levels observed in animal models and human studies. Cannabinoid receptor agonists, such as delta-9-tetrahydrocannabinol (THC) and cannabidiol (CBD), may offer therapeutic benefit in cluster headaches by modulating pain processing and neuroinflammation.

Nitric Oxide (NO):

Nitric oxide (NO) is a signaling molecule involved in vasodilation, neurotransmission, and inflammation. Dysregulation of the nitric oxide system has been implicated in the pathophysiology of cluster headaches, with elevated levels of NO observed during headache attacks. Nitric oxide synthase (NOS) inhibitors, such as L-arginine analogs, may offer therapeutic benefit in cluster headaches by reducing NO production and vasodilation in the cranial vasculature.

Conclusion:

Neurotransmitters and neuromodulators play a crucial role in the pathophysiology of cluster headaches by mediating pain transmission, modulating neuronal excitability, and regulating autonomic function. Dysregulation of these signaling molecules may contribute to the generation and propagation of headache attacks and represent potential targets for novel therapeutic interventions. By elucidating the roles of neurotransmitters and neuromodulators in cluster headaches, researchers can advance our understanding of this debilitating condition and develop more effective treatments aimed at alleviating pain and improving patient outcomes.

CHAPTER 3: PATHOPHYSIOLOGY OF CLUSTER HEADACHES

Trigeminal Nociceptive Pathways

The trigeminal nociceptive pathways play a central role in the transmission of pain signals originating from the face and head to the brain. Understanding the intricate anatomy and physiology of these pathways is essential for unraveling the mechanisms underlying cluster headaches and developing targeted therapeutic interventions. This subchapter provides a comprehensive exploration of the trigeminal nociceptive pathways, highlighting their organization, neurotransmitter signaling, and role in the pathophysiology of cluster headaches.

Anatomy of the Trigeminal Nerve:

The trigeminal nerve (CN V) is the fifth cranial nerve and is responsible for transmitting sensory information from the face, oral cavity, and head to the brain. It consists of three main branches: the ophthalmic nerve (V1), the maxillary nerve (V2), and the mandibular nerve (V3). These branches innervate different regions of the face and transmit sensory signals related to touch, temperature, and pain.

Trigeminal Ganglion:

The cell bodies of sensory neurons of the trigeminal nerve are located in the trigeminal ganglion, which is situated within the middle cranial fossa. The trigeminal ganglion serves as a relay station for sensory input from the face and sends projections to various regions of the brainstem, including the spinal trigeminal nucleus and the trigeminal nucleus caudalis.

Central Trigeminal Pathways:

The central trigeminal pathways encompass a network of ascending and descending fibers that transmit sensory information from the trigeminal nerve to higher centers in the brain. These pathways consist of three main nuclei within the brainstem: the spinal trigeminal nucleus, the principal sensory nucleus, and the mesencephalic nucleus. Each nucleus receives input from different branches of the trigeminal nerve and contributes to the processing and modulation of sensory signals.

1. **Spinal Trigeminal Nucleus (SpV):** The spinal trigeminal nucleus is located in the medulla oblongata and is divided into three subnuclei: oral, interpolar, and caudal. It receives nociceptive input from the face and head via the ophthalmic, maxillary, and mandibular divisions of the trigeminal nerve. The SpV plays a crucial role in transmitting nociceptive signals to higher brain centers and mediating the perception of pain.
2. **Principal Sensory Nucleus (PSN):** The principal sensory nucleus is located in the pons and receives tactile and proprioceptive input from the face via the trigeminal nerve. It plays a role in processing non-nociceptive sensory information and integrating it with nociceptive signals from the SpV.

3. **Mesencephalic Nucleus (MesV):** The mesencephalic nucleus is located in the midbrain and receives proprioceptive input from the muscles of mastication via the mandibular division of the trigeminal nerve. It plays a role in proprioception and reflexive responses to jaw movement.

Neurotransmitter Signaling:

Neurotransmitters play a key role in mediating synaptic transmission within the trigeminal nociceptive pathways. Glutamate is the primary excitatory neurotransmitter involved in transmitting sensory signals from the trigeminal nerve to the brainstem nuclei. GABA (gamma-aminobutyric acid) is the primary inhibitory neurotransmitter that modulates neuronal excitability and synaptic transmission within the trigeminal nuclei. Other neurotransmitters, such as serotonin, dopamine, and neuropeptides like substance P and CGRP, also play a modulatory role in pain processing and nociceptive signaling within the trigeminal pathways.

Role in Cluster Headaches:

The trigeminal nociceptive pathways are believed to play a central role in the pathophysiology of cluster headaches. Activation of nociceptive fibers within the trigeminal nerve leads to the transmission of pain signals to the brainstem nuclei, resulting in the perception of headache pain. Additionally, sensitization of trigeminal neurons and dysregulation of neurotransmitter signaling may contribute to the development and maintenance of cluster headaches.

Therapeutic Implications:

Targeting the trigeminal nociceptive pathways represents a promising therapeutic strategy for the management of cluster headaches. Pharmacological agents that modulate neurotransmitter signaling, such as triptans (5-HT1B/1D receptor agonists) and CGRP antagonists, have shown efficacy in aborting cluster headache attacks by inhibiting nociceptive transmission within the trigeminal pathways. Additionally, neuromodulation techniques, such as occipital nerve stimulation or deep brain stimulation, may modulate activity within the trigeminal nuclei and alleviate symptoms in refractory cases.

Conclusion:

The trigeminal nociceptive pathways play a central role in the transmission of pain signals from the face and head to the brain. Dysfunction of these pathways may contribute to the pathophysiology of cluster headaches, leading to the perception of headache pain and associated symptoms. By elucidating the anatomy, neurotransmitter signaling, and role of the trigeminal nociceptive pathways in cluster headaches, researchers can advance our understanding of this debilitating condition and develop more effective treatments aimed at alleviating pain and improving patient outcomes.

Vascular Mechanisms and Vasodilation

Vascular mechanisms and vasodilation play a significant role in the pathophysiology of cluster headaches, contributing to the throbbing pain and autonomic symptoms characteristic of this condition. Understanding the intricate interplay between vascular changes, neurogenic inflammation, and pain signaling is essential for unraveling the mechanisms underlying cluster headaches. This subchapter delves into the vascular mechanisms and vasodilation involved in cluster headaches, exploring their impact on pain perception and potential therapeutic interventions.

Vascular Anatomy of the Head and Neck:

The head and neck are richly vascularized regions supplied by branches of the external and internal carotid arteries. The cranial vasculature includes arteries such as the middle meningeal artery, anterior cerebral artery, and posterior cerebral artery, which supply blood to the brain and meninges. The extracranial vasculature includes branches of the external carotid artery, such as the superficial temporal artery and maxillary artery, which supply blood to the face, scalp, and deep structures of the head.

Role of Vasodilation in Cluster Headaches:

Vasodilation is a hallmark feature of cluster headaches and is believed to contribute to the throbbing pain and autonomic symptoms experienced during attacks. Several mechanisms may underlie vasodilation in cluster headaches:

1. **Neurogenic Inflammation:** Activation of trigeminal nociceptive pathways leads to the release of neuropeptides such as calcitonin gene-related peptide (CGRP) and substance P, which promote vasodilation and neurogenic inflammation in the cranial vasculature. Vasodilation may be mediated by direct effects on vascular smooth muscle cells or through the activation of endothelial cells and release of vasodilatory factors.
2. **Nitric Oxide (NO) Pathway:** Nitric oxide (NO) is a potent vasodilator produced by endothelial cells in response to various stimuli, including neurotransmitter release and shear stress. Dysregulation of the NO pathway has been implicated in cluster headaches, with elevated levels of NO observed during headache attacks. NO-mediated vasodilation may contribute to the dilation of cranial blood vessels and the pulsatile nature of cluster headache pain.
3. **Autonomic Dysregulation:** Dysfunction of the autonomic nervous system, particularly the parasympathetic division, may lead to aberrant vasodilatory responses

in cluster headaches. Parasympathetic activation can promote vasodilation through the release of acetylcholine and activation of muscarinic receptors on vascular smooth muscle cells.

Vascular Responses During Cluster Headache Attacks:

During cluster headache attacks, there is evidence of vascular changes in the cranial circulation, including:

1. **Arterial Dilation:** Imaging studies have demonstrated dilation of intracranial and extracranial arteries during cluster headache attacks, particularly in the ipsilateral hemisphere. This dilation may be mediated by neurogenic mechanisms, involving the release of vasodilatory neuropeptides from trigeminal nociceptive fibers.
2. **Increased Blood Flow:** Doppler ultrasound studies have shown increased blood flow velocity in the middle cerebral artery during cluster headache attacks, reflecting increased cerebral perfusion. This hyperperfusion may contribute to the pulsatile nature of cluster headache pain and the associated throbbing sensation.
3. **Cutaneous Vasodilation:** Autonomic symptoms such as facial flushing and nasal congestion are indicative of cutaneous vasodilation during cluster headache attacks. Activation of trigeminal-autonomic reflex pathways may lead to the release of vasodilatory neuropeptides, causing dilation of blood vessels in the face and scalp.

Therapeutic Implications:

Targeting vascular mechanisms and vasodilation represents a potential therapeutic strategy for the management of cluster headaches. Pharmacological agents that modulate vascular tone or inhibit vasodilation may offer relief from headache symptoms. Triptans, which act as serotonin agonists and constrict cranial blood vessels, are effective in aborting cluster headache attacks by reversing vasodilation and reducing neurogenic inflammation. Additionally, CGRP antagonists block the vasodilatory effects of CGRP and have shown efficacy in preventing cluster headache attacks.

Conclusion:

Vascular mechanisms and vasodilation play a significant role in the pathophysiology of cluster headaches, contributing to the throbbing pain and autonomic symptoms characteristic of this condition. Neurogenic inflammation, nitric oxide-mediated vasodilation, and autonomic dysregulation are key mechanisms underlying vasodilatory responses during cluster headache attacks. Understanding these vascular mechanisms provides insights into potential therapeutic targets for the management of cluster headaches, with pharmacological agents aimed at modulating vascular tone and inhibiting vasodilation showing promise in clinical practice.

Inflammatory Mediators and Neurogenic Inflammation

Inflammatory mediators and neurogenic inflammation play a pivotal role in the pathophysiology of cluster headaches, contributing to the initiation, propagation, and maintenance of pain signals. Understanding the intricate interplay between inflammatory mediators, neurogenic inflammation, and pain pathways is crucial for unraveling the mechanisms underlying cluster headaches. This subchapter provides an in-depth exploration of the inflammatory mediators and neurogenic inflammation involved in cluster headaches, shedding light on their role in pain perception and potential therapeutic interventions.

Inflammatory Mediators:

Inflammatory mediators are signaling molecules produced in response to tissue injury, infection, or immune activation. In the context of cluster headaches, several inflammatory mediators have been implicated in the generation and modulation of pain signals:

1. **Calcitonin Gene-Related Peptide (CGRP):** CGRP is a potent vasodilator and neuropeptide released from trigeminal sensory neurons in response to nociceptive stimuli. Elevated levels of CGRP have been observed during cluster headache attacks, and CGRP receptor antagonists have shown efficacy in aborting attacks and preventing their recurrence.
2. **Substance P:** Substance P is a neuropeptide involved in pain transmission and neurogenic inflammation. Trigeminal sensory neurons release substance P in response to noxious stimuli, contributing to vasodilation and plasma extravasation in the cranial vasculature.
3. **Bradykinin:** Bradykinin is a peptide released from damaged tissues and contributes to pain sensation and inflammation by activating bradykinin receptors on sensory neurons. Increased levels of bradykinin have been detected in the saliva of cluster headache patients during attacks.
4. **Prostaglandins:** Prostaglandins are lipid mediators produced from arachidonic acid metabolism and contribute to inflammation, pain, and vasodilation. Cyclooxygenase (COX) enzymes catalyze the synthesis of prostaglandins, and nonsteroidal anti-inflammatory drugs (NSAIDs) that inhibit COX activity may provide relief from cluster headache pain.

Neurogenic Inflammation:

Neurogenic inflammation refers to the inflammatory response initiated by the release of neuropeptides from sensory nerve fibers, particularly from trigeminal nociceptive fibers, in response to noxious stimuli. Key features of neurogenic inflammation in cluster headaches include:

1. **Vasodilation:** Neuropeptides such as CGRP and substance P promote vasodilation by acting on vascular smooth muscle cells and endothelial cells, leading to increased blood flow and plasma extravasation in the cranial vasculature.
2. **Plasma Extravasation:** Neurogenic inflammation results in the leakage of plasma proteins, such as albumin and fibrinogen, from blood vessels into the surrounding tissues. This extravasation contributes to tissue edema, inflammation, and sensitization of nociceptive neurons.
3. **Immune Cell Recruitment:** Neuropeptides released during neurogenic inflammation can recruit immune cells, such as neutrophils and mast cells, to the site of inflammation. These immune cells release pro-inflammatory cytokines and mediators, amplifying the inflammatory response and contributing to pain sensitization.

Role in Cluster Headaches:

Neurogenic inflammation plays a central role in the pathophysiology of cluster headaches, contributing to the generation and propagation of pain signals. Several lines of evidence support the involvement of inflammatory mediators and neurogenic inflammation in cluster headaches:

1. **Elevated Levels of Inflammatory Mediators:** Studies have demonstrated elevated levels of CGRP, substance P, bradykinin, and prostaglandins in cluster headache patients during attacks, suggesting a role for these mediators in pain generation and vasodilation.
2. **Peripheral Sensitization:** Neurogenic inflammation can induce peripheral sensitization of nociceptive neurons,

lowering their activation threshold and increasing their responsiveness to stimuli. This sensitization may contribute to the hyperalgesia and allodynia experienced by cluster headache patients during attacks.
3. **Central Sensitization:** Prolonged activation of nociceptive pathways by neurogenic inflammation can lead to central sensitization, a process characterized by enhanced synaptic transmission and amplification of pain signals within the central nervous system. Central sensitization may contribute to the chronicity and severity of cluster headaches.

Therapeutic Implications:

Targeting inflammatory mediators and neurogenic inflammation represents a potential therapeutic strategy for the management of cluster headaches. Pharmacological agents that inhibit the release or activity of neuropeptides, such as CGRP antagonists, substance P receptor antagonists, and bradykinin receptor antagonists, may offer relief from headache pain and autonomic symptoms. Additionally, anti-inflammatory agents such as NSAIDs and corticosteroids may attenuate neurogenic inflammation and provide symptomatic relief in acute attacks.

Conclusion:

Inflammatory mediators and neurogenic inflammation play a critical role in the pathophysiology of cluster headaches, contributing to pain generation, vasodilation, and sensitization of nociceptive pathways. By elucidating the mechanisms underlying inflammatory processes in cluster headaches, researchers can identify novel therapeutic targets aimed at modulating neurogenic inflammation and alleviating pain and associated symptoms. Integration of anti-inflammatory strategies with existing treatment approaches may offer improved management options for individuals suffering from cluster headaches.

Role of Central Sensitization

Central sensitization is a fundamental neurophysiological process implicated in the pathophysiology of cluster headaches, contributing to the amplification and maintenance of pain signals within the central nervous system. Understanding the mechanisms underlying central sensitization is essential for unraveling the complexities of cluster headaches and developing targeted therapeutic interventions. This subchapter explores the role of central sensitization in cluster headaches, highlighting its impact on pain perception, neuroplasticity, and potential treatment strategies.

Definition of Central Sensitization:

Central sensitization refers to the amplification of nociceptive signals within the central nervous system, leading to heightened pain sensitivity and prolonged pain responses. It is characterized by increased excitability of nociceptive neurons, alterations in synaptic transmission, and neuroplastic changes within pain-processing circuits. Central sensitization can occur in response to persistent nociceptive input, neuroinflammation, or dysfunction of inhibitory pain modulatory pathways.

Mechanisms of Central Sensitization:

Several mechanisms contribute to the development and maintenance of central sensitization in cluster headaches:

1. **Nociceptive Input:** Persistent activation of trigeminal nociceptive pathways by nociceptive stimuli, such as inflammation or tissue injury, leads to the release of excitatory neurotransmitters and neuropeptides within the central nervous system. This sustained input triggers neuroplastic changes in pain-processing circuits,

including the spinal cord, brainstem, and higher cortical regions.
2. **Glutamatergic Transmission:** Glutamate is the primary excitatory neurotransmitter involved in nociceptive signaling and synaptic transmission within the central nervous system. Excessive release of glutamate and activation of N-methyl-D-aspartate (NMDA) receptors contribute to synaptic potentiation, long-term potentiation (LTP), and hyperexcitability of nociceptive neurons, resulting in central sensitization.
3. **Neuroinflammation:** Neurogenic inflammation and the release of pro-inflammatory cytokines and mediators contribute to neuroinflammatory processes within the central nervous system. These inflammatory molecules sensitize nociceptive neurons, promote synaptic plasticity, and facilitate the development of central sensitization.
4. **Descending Modulatory Pathways:** Dysfunction of descending modulatory pathways, including the endogenous pain inhibitory system and descending facilitatory pathways, can contribute to the development of central sensitization. Imbalance between inhibitory and facilitatory influences on nociceptive neurons may result in enhanced pain transmission and sensitization.

Impact of Central Sensitization on Pain Perception:

Central sensitization plays a crucial role in shaping pain perception and contributing to the clinical features of cluster headaches:

1. **Hyperalgesia:** Central sensitization leads to an exaggerated response to noxious stimuli, resulting in hyperalgesia, or increased pain sensitivity. Cluster headache patients may experience heightened pain intensity and duration during attacks due to central sensitization processes.

2. **Allodynia:** Central sensitization can also lead to the perception of pain in response to non-noxious stimuli, a phenomenon known as allodynia. Cutaneous allodynia, characterized by pain in response to light touch or pressure, is commonly observed in cluster headache patients during attacks.
3. **Temporal Summation:** Central sensitization results in temporal summation of pain, whereby repetitive or prolonged stimulation of nociceptive pathways leads to an increasing perception of pain over time. This phenomenon contributes to the progressive escalation of pain intensity during cluster headache attacks.

Neuroplastic Changes in Central Sensitization:

Central sensitization is associated with neuroplastic changes within pain-processing circuits, including alterations in synaptic strength, neuronal excitability, and connectivity:

1. **Synaptic Potentiation:** Enhanced synaptic transmission and potentiation of excitatory synapses contribute to the amplification of nociceptive signals within the central nervous system. This synaptic plasticity underlies the persistence of pain and the development of chronic pain states in cluster headache patients.
2. **Neuronal Hyperexcitability:** Central sensitization leads to increased neuronal excitability and reduced threshold for activation of nociceptive neurons. This hyperexcitability contributes to spontaneous pain, evoked pain responses, and sensitization of pain pathways in cluster headache patients.
3. **Neurogenesis and Rewiring:** Central sensitization is associated with structural and functional changes in pain-processing regions of the brain, including alterations in neuronal morphology, synaptic connectivity, and neurogenesis. These neuroplastic changes contribute to

the maladaptive remodeling of pain circuits and the establishment of chronic pain states.

Therapeutic Implications:

Targeting central sensitization represents a promising therapeutic strategy for the management of cluster headaches. Pharmacological agents that modulate glutamatergic transmission, such as NMDA receptor antagonists, may attenuate central sensitization and reduce pain intensity. Additionally, neuromodulation techniques, including transcranial magnetic stimulation (TMS) and transcutaneous electrical nerve stimulation (TENS), may modulate excitability within pain-processing circuits and alleviate symptoms in cluster headache patients.

Conclusion:

Central sensitization is a key neurophysiological process implicated in the pathophysiology of cluster headaches, contributing to heightened pain sensitivity, neuroplastic changes, and the maintenance of pain states. By elucidating the mechanisms underlying central sensitization, researchers can identify novel therapeutic targets and develop more effective treatment strategies aimed at alleviating pain and improving patient outcomes in cluster headache management. Integration of central sensitization-targeted therapies with existing treatment approaches holds promise for optimizing the management of this debilitating condition.

Genetic and Environmental Factors

Genetic and environmental factors play pivotal roles in the etiology and pathogenesis of cluster headaches, influencing susceptibility, symptomatology, and disease progression.

Understanding the complex interplay between genetic predisposition and environmental triggers is essential for elucidating the mechanisms underlying cluster headaches. This subchapter provides an in-depth exploration of the genetic and environmental factors associated with cluster headaches, shedding light on their contributions to disease development and potential therapeutic implications.

Genetic Factors:

1. **Familial Aggregation:** Cluster headaches exhibit familial aggregation, with a higher prevalence of the condition among first-degree relatives of affected individuals compared to the general population. Genetic studies have identified familial clusters of cluster headache cases, suggesting a genetic predisposition to the condition.
2. **Candidate Genes:** Genome-wide association studies (GWAS) and candidate gene approaches have identified several genetic variants associated with cluster headaches. These include variants in genes encoding receptors, ion channels, neuropeptides, and neurotransmitter transporters involved in pain processing, vasomotor regulation, and circadian rhythms.
3. **Hypothalamic Involvement:** Genetic studies have implicated genes involved in hypothalamic function and circadian rhythm regulation in the pathogenesis of cluster headaches. Disruptions in the expression or function of these genes may contribute to the dysregulation of the hypothalamus observed in cluster headache patients.
4. **Serotonergic System:** Genes encoding components of the serotonergic system, including serotonin receptors and transporters, have been implicated in cluster headaches. Alterations in serotonin signaling may modulate pain sensitivity, vasomotor tone, and autonomic function, contributing to the pathophysiology of cluster headaches.

Environmental Factors:

1. **Triggers and Precipitants:** Various environmental factors can trigger or precipitate cluster headache attacks, including alcohol consumption, cigarette smoking, high-altitude exposure, and changes in sleep patterns. Identifying and avoiding these triggers may help manage cluster headache symptoms and reduce the frequency and severity of attacks.
2. **Seasonal Variations:** Cluster headaches often exhibit seasonal variations, with higher prevalence during certain times of the year. Environmental factors such as changes in temperature, humidity, and daylight hours may influence disease activity and symptom onset in susceptible individuals.
3. **Occupational Exposures:** Occupational exposures to chemicals, pollutants, and allergens have been implicated as potential triggers for cluster headaches. Individuals working in certain industries or environments may be at increased risk of developing cluster headaches due to exposure to specific substances or environmental factors.
4. **Psychosocial Stress:** Psychosocial stressors, including work-related stress, family conflicts, and life events, can exacerbate cluster headache symptoms and increase disease burden. Stress management techniques, relaxation therapies, and psychological interventions may help alleviate symptoms and improve quality of life in cluster headache patients.

Gene-Environment Interactions:

1. **Gene-Environment Interplay:** Genetic susceptibility to cluster headaches may interact with environmental factors to modulate disease risk and phenotype. Gene-environment interactions may influence susceptibility to

triggers, disease severity, treatment response, and disease progression in cluster headache patients.
2. **Epigenetic Modifications:** Epigenetic mechanisms, including DNA methylation, histone modification, and non-coding RNA regulation, may mediate the effects of environmental factors on gene expression and phenotype in cluster headache patients. Epigenetic modifications may serve as molecular links between genetic predisposition and environmental exposures in the pathogenesis of cluster headaches.

Therapeutic Implications:

1. **Personalized Medicine:** Understanding the genetic and environmental determinants of cluster headaches may enable personalized approaches to treatment and management. Genetic profiling and identification of environmental triggers could help tailor therapeutic interventions to individual patients, optimizing treatment outcomes and minimizing adverse effects.
2. **Targeted Interventions:** Targeting specific genetic pathways or environmental triggers implicated in cluster headaches may offer novel therapeutic avenues for disease management. Pharmacological agents that modulate serotonergic signaling, vasomotor regulation, or hypothalamic function may be effective in treating cluster headaches in genetically susceptible individuals.
3. **Lifestyle Modifications:** Lifestyle modifications, including avoidance of known triggers, adoption of healthy sleep habits, and stress management techniques, may help reduce the frequency and severity of cluster headache attacks. Identifying and addressing environmental factors contributing to disease onset or exacerbation is an integral part of comprehensive cluster headache management.

Conclusion:

Genetic and environmental factors play critical roles in the etiology and pathogenesis of cluster headaches, influencing disease susceptibility, symptomatology, and treatment response. Elucidating the complex interplay between genetic predisposition and environmental triggers is essential for understanding the mechanisms underlying cluster headaches and developing targeted therapeutic interventions. Integration of genetic and environmental factors into clinical practice may facilitate personalized approaches to treatment and management, ultimately improving outcomes for individuals

CHAPTER 4: CLINICAL PRESENTATION AND DIAGNOSIS

Symptomatology and Diagnostic Criteria

Cluster headaches represent one of the most excruciating and debilitating primary headache disorders, characterized by intense, unilateral pain accompanied by autonomic symptoms. Understanding the symptomatology and diagnostic criteria of cluster headaches is paramount for accurate diagnosis, timely intervention, and effective management. This subchapter delves into the intricate manifestations of cluster headaches, elucidates the diagnostic criteria outlined by expert consensus, and discusses the challenges involved in distinguishing cluster headaches from other headache disorders.

Clinical Manifestations:

1. **Severe Unilateral Pain:** The hallmark symptom of cluster headaches is severe, unilateral pain, typically centered around the eye, temple, or forehead. Described as excruciating, stabbing, or burning, this pain often reaches its peak intensity within minutes of onset. Patients may describe it as the worst pain they have ever experienced.

2. **Short Duration Attacks:** Cluster headache attacks are characterized by their relatively short duration, ranging from 15 minutes to 3 hours. Despite their brevity, the intensity of pain can be debilitating, leading to significant distress and impairment in daily functioning. The cyclical nature of attacks, occurring in clusters or bouts, distinguishes cluster headaches from other headache disorders.
3. **Autonomic Symptoms:** One of the defining features of cluster headaches is the presence of ipsilateral autonomic symptoms. These include lacrimation (tearing), conjunctival injection (redness of the eye), nasal congestion or rhinorrhea (runny nose), ptosis (drooping eyelid), and miosis (constricted pupil). These autonomic manifestations often accompany the pain and contribute to the characteristic clinical presentation of cluster headaches.
4. **Restlessness and Agitation:** During cluster headache attacks, patients may exhibit restlessness, agitation, or a sense of unease. They may pace, rock back and forth, or engage in repetitive movements in an attempt to alleviate the pain. This restlessness is a distinctive feature of cluster headaches and may help differentiate them from other headache disorders.

Diagnostic Criteria:

1. **International Classification of Headache Disorders (ICHD):** The International Classification of Headache Disorders (ICHD) provides the most widely accepted diagnostic criteria for cluster headaches. According to the latest edition (ICHD-3), the diagnostic criteria for cluster headaches include:
    - At least five attacks fulfilling criteria B-D
    - Severe or very severe unilateral orbital, supraorbital, or temporal pain lasting 15-180

minutes
- At least one of the following autonomic features ipsilateral to the headache:
  - Conjunctival injection and/or lacrimation
  - Nasal congestion and/or rhinorrhea
  - Eyelid edema and/or forehead and facial sweating
  - Pupillary constriction and/or ptosis
- Attacks have a frequency of 1 every other day to 8 per day
- Attacks occur in clusters lasting for weeks to months followed by spontaneous remission periods lasting months to years
- The headache is not better accounted for by another ICHD-3 diagnosis

2. **Clinical Evaluation:** Diagnosis of cluster headaches primarily relies on a thorough clinical evaluation, including a detailed history of headache characteristics, associated symptoms, and temporal patterns of attacks. Neurological examination may reveal autonomic signs consistent with cluster headaches, supporting the diagnosis.

3. **Exclusion of Secondary Causes:** It is crucial to rule out secondary causes of headache through appropriate diagnostic testing, such as neuroimaging (e.g., magnetic resonance imaging, computed tomography) and laboratory investigations. Secondary headaches with features resembling cluster headaches, such as those due to intracranial pathology or substance use, must be excluded.

Challenges in Diagnosis:

1. **Overlap with Other Headache Disorders:** Cluster headaches may share clinical features with other primary headache disorders, such as migraine, trigeminal

autonomic cephalalgias (TACs), and paroxysmal hemicrania. Distinguishing between these disorders can be challenging, particularly during the early stages of evaluation.
2. **Variability in Presentation:** The presentation of cluster headaches can vary widely among individuals and across episodes. Some patients may not exhibit typical autonomic symptoms, while others may experience atypical features or comorbidities that complicate the diagnosis.
3. **Diagnostic Delay:** Due to the relatively low prevalence of cluster headaches and the lack of awareness among healthcare providers, there is often a significant delay in diagnosis. Patients may undergo multiple consultations and diagnostic tests before receiving a definitive diagnosis, leading to unnecessary suffering and frustration.

Conclusion:

Symptomatology and diagnostic criteria are fundamental aspects of understanding and diagnosing cluster headaches. Recognition of the hallmark features, including severe unilateral pain, autonomic symptoms, and episodic clustering, is essential for accurate diagnosis and initiation of appropriate treatment. By adhering to established diagnostic criteria and considering the challenges involved in distinguishing cluster headaches from other headache disorders, healthcare providers can provide timely intervention and improve outcomes for patients affected by this debilitating condition. Continued education and awareness efforts are essential to reduce diagnostic delays and ensure that individuals with cluster headaches receive prompt and effective management.

Differential Diagnosis

Differential diagnosis is a critical aspect of evaluating patients with suspected cluster headaches, as several primary and secondary headache disorders may present with overlapping clinical features. Distinguishing cluster headaches from other conditions is essential for appropriate management and treatment selection. This subchapter explores the differential diagnosis of cluster headaches, highlighting key distinguishing features and diagnostic considerations for commonly encountered headache disorders.

1. Migraine:

- **Clinical Features:** Migraine headaches typically present with unilateral or bilateral throbbing pain, often accompanied by nausea, vomiting, photophobia, and phonophobia. Attacks may last from a few hours to several days and are commonly preceded by aura symptoms in some patients.
- **Distinguishing Features:** Unlike cluster headaches, migraines usually have longer attack durations, associated symptoms like nausea and photophobia, and a pulsating quality to the pain. Additionally, migraines do not exhibit the same pattern of episodic clustering seen in cluster headaches.

2. Trigeminal Autonomic Cephalalgias (TACs):

- **Clinical Features:** TACs, including paroxysmal hemicrania and hemicrania continua, share some similarities with cluster headaches, such as unilateral head pain and autonomic symptoms. However, they differ in attack duration, frequency, and response to treatment.
- **Distinguishing Features:** Paroxysmal hemicrania, for example, presents with shorter and more frequent attacks than cluster headaches, often responsive to indomethacin. Hemicrania continua presents with continuous unilateral

pain, with superimposed exacerbations responsive to indomethacin.

3. Trigeminal Neuralgia:

- **Clinical Features:** Trigeminal neuralgia is characterized by severe, lancinating facial pain along the distribution of the trigeminal nerve, often triggered by light touch or movement. Attacks are brief, lasting seconds to minutes, and may occur in clusters.
- **Distinguishing Features:** Unlike cluster headaches, trigeminal neuralgia pain is strictly unilateral and typically does not involve autonomic symptoms or exhibit the same episodic clustering pattern. Imaging studies may be necessary to rule out structural lesions compressing the trigeminal nerve.

4. Tension-Type Headache:

- **Clinical Features:** Tension-type headaches present with bilateral, pressing or tightening head pain that is typically mild to moderate in intensity. Unlike cluster headaches, tension-type headaches do not exhibit autonomic symptoms and are not associated with the same level of disability.
- **Distinguishing Features:** The absence of autonomic symptoms, the bilateral distribution of pain, and the lack of episodic clustering help differentiate tension-type headaches from cluster headaches.

5. Secondary Headaches:

- **Clinical Features:** Secondary headaches can mimic the presentation of primary headache disorders, including cluster headaches. Causes may include intracranial pathology (e.g., tumors, hemorrhage), vascular disorders (e.g., arterial dissection, arteritis), or substance use (e.g.,

medication overuse headache, substance withdrawal).
- **Distinguishing Features:** Secondary headaches often present with atypical features, such as sudden onset, progressive worsening, neurological deficits, or associated systemic symptoms. Diagnostic imaging and laboratory investigations are essential for identifying underlying causes and ruling out secondary headaches.

Conclusion: Differential diagnosis is essential in evaluating patients with suspected cluster headaches to ensure accurate diagnosis and appropriate management. Understanding the distinguishing features of cluster headaches compared to other primary headache disorders, such as migraine and trigeminal autonomic cephalalgias, as well as recognizing red flags for secondary headaches, is critical for guiding clinical decision-making. A thorough clinical evaluation, including history-taking, physical examination, and targeted investigations, is necessary to arrive at the correct diagnosis and provide optimal care for patients with headache disorders.

Diagnostic Imaging Techniques

Diagnostic imaging plays a crucial role in the evaluation of patients with suspected cluster headaches, particularly in ruling out secondary causes and identifying structural abnormalities that may contribute to headache symptoms. While cluster headaches are primarily diagnosed based on clinical criteria, imaging studies can provide valuable information to support the diagnosis and guide treatment decisions. This subchapter examines the role of various diagnostic imaging techniques in the assessment of cluster headaches, highlighting their indications, advantages, and limitations.

1. Magnetic Resonance Imaging (MRI):

- **Indications:** MRI is the preferred imaging modality for evaluating patients with suspected cluster headaches, particularly to rule out secondary causes such as intracranial lesions, vascular abnormalities, or inflammatory conditions.
- **Advantages:** MRI offers excellent soft tissue contrast and multiplanar imaging capabilities, allowing for detailed visualization of intracranial structures, including the brain, blood vessels, and cranial nerves.
- **Limitations:** While MRI is highly sensitive for detecting structural abnormalities, it may not always reveal specific findings in patients with primary headache disorders like cluster headaches. False-positive findings and incidentalomas are relatively common, necessitating careful interpretation of imaging findings in the context of clinical presentation.

2. Computed Tomography (CT):

- **Indications:** CT may be used in the acute setting to rule out emergent causes of headache, such as intracranial hemorrhage or acute stroke, particularly when MRI is not readily available or contraindicated.
- **Advantages:** CT is widely available, quick to perform, and well-suited for detecting acute hemorrhage or bony abnormalities. It is particularly useful in emergency situations requiring rapid assessment.
- **Limitations:** CT has lower sensitivity for detecting soft tissue abnormalities compared to MRI and involves exposure to ionizing radiation, which may limit its utility for repeated or long-term imaging surveillance.

3. Magnetic Resonance Angiography (MRA):

- **Indications:** MRA is indicated when evaluating patients with suspected vascular causes of headache, such as

arterial dissection, arteriovenous malformations (AVMs), or intracranial aneurysms.
- **Advantages:** MRA provides non-invasive visualization of intracranial blood vessels, offering detailed assessment of vascular anatomy and detecting abnormalities such as stenosis, aneurysms, or vascular malformations.
- **Limitations:** MRA may have limited spatial resolution compared to conventional angiography techniques and may not always provide sufficient detail for precise characterization of vascular lesions. Additionally, it may not be suitable for patients with contraindications to MRI, such as those with implanted metallic devices.

4. Positron Emission Tomography (PET):

- **Indications:** PET imaging may be utilized in research settings to investigate functional changes in the brain associated with cluster headaches, such as alterations in regional cerebral blood flow, glucose metabolism, or neurotransmitter activity.
- **Advantages:** PET allows for quantitative assessment of physiological processes within the brain, providing insights into underlying pathophysiological mechanisms of cluster headaches.
- **Limitations:** PET imaging is not routinely used in clinical practice for diagnosing or managing cluster headaches due to limited availability, high cost, and technical complexity. It is primarily employed in research studies and may not be accessible to all patients.

5. Functional MRI (fMRI):

- **Indications:** fMRI is used to study brain function and connectivity patterns in patients with cluster headaches, providing insights into neural networks involved in pain processing, autonomic regulation, and response to

treatment.
- **Advantages:** fMRI offers non-invasive assessment of brain activity during headache attacks or interictal periods, facilitating the identification of aberrant functional connectivity and neural correlates of cluster headaches.
- **Limitations:** fMRI requires specialized equipment and expertise, limiting its availability and applicability in routine clinical practice. Interpretation of fMRI findings may be challenging due to variability in study protocols and analytical techniques.

Conclusion: Diagnostic imaging techniques play a valuable role in the evaluation of patients with suspected cluster headaches, aiding in the identification of secondary causes, characterization of structural abnormalities, and investigation of underlying pathophysiological mechanisms. While MRI remains the imaging modality of choice for comprehensive assessment, other techniques such as CT, MRA, PET, and fMRI may be selectively employed based on clinical indications and availability. Collaborative multidisciplinary approaches involving neurologists, radiologists, and headache specialists are essential for optimal utilization and interpretation of diagnostic imaging studies in the management of cluster headaches.

Role of Biomarkers and Genetic Testing

Biomarkers and genetic testing have emerged as promising avenues for advancing the understanding, diagnosis, and management of cluster headaches. These tools offer insights into the underlying pathophysiological mechanisms, identify potential genetic predispositions, and facilitate personalized approaches to treatment. This subchapter explores the evolving role of biomarkers and genetic testing in the context of cluster headaches, highlighting their potential applications, challenges, and future directions.

1. Biomarkers in Cluster Headaches:

Biomarkers are measurable indicators that reflect physiological or pathological processes associated with a disease. In the context of cluster headaches, biomarkers may include biochemical, neuroimaging, or genetic markers that provide objective measures of disease activity, severity, or treatment response.

- **Biochemical Biomarkers:** Studies have identified potential biochemical biomarkers associated with cluster headaches, including markers of inflammation, oxidative stress, and neurotransmitter imbalance. These biomarkers may offer insights into underlying pathophysiological mechanisms and aid in the development of targeted therapeutic interventions.
- **Neuroimaging Biomarkers:** Advanced neuroimaging techniques, such as functional MRI (fMRI) and positron emission tomography (PET), can identify neuroanatomical and functional alterations in the brain associated with cluster headaches. Biomarkers derived from neuroimaging data may help elucidate aberrant neural circuits, identify treatment targets, and monitor disease progression.
- **Genetic Biomarkers:** Genetic variations associated with cluster headaches may serve as potential biomarkers for disease susceptibility, phenotype expression, and treatment response. Genome-wide association studies (GWAS) and candidate gene approaches have identified genetic loci and polymorphisms implicated in cluster headaches, offering insights into the genetic basis of the disorder.

2. Genetic Testing in Cluster Headaches:

Genetic testing allows for the identification of specific genetic variants or mutations associated with cluster headaches, offering opportunities for personalized risk assessment, diagnosis, and treatment optimization. While genetic testing for cluster headaches is still in its infancy, ongoing research efforts hold promise for expanding its clinical utility.

- **Candidate Gene Testing:** Candidate gene studies have identified potential genetic candidates involved in the pathogenesis of cluster headaches, including genes encoding neuropeptides, neurotransmitter receptors, and ion channels implicated in pain processing, vasomotor regulation, and circadian rhythms. Targeted genetic testing of these candidate genes may help identify individuals at increased risk of developing cluster headaches and guide treatment decisions.
- **Genome-Wide Association Studies (GWAS):** GWAS leverage high-throughput genotyping technologies to scan the entire genome for genetic variants associated with cluster headaches. By analyzing large cohorts of patients with cluster headaches and healthy controls, GWAS can identify novel genetic loci and pathways implicated in the disorder, paving the way for precision medicine approaches.

Challenges and Future Directions:

Despite the potential benefits of biomarkers and genetic testing in cluster headaches, several challenges must be addressed to realize their full clinical impact.

- **Validation and Replication:** Biomarkers and genetic variants identified in research studies require validation and replication in independent cohorts to ensure their reliability and reproducibility across different populations.
- **Clinical Translation:** Biomarkers and genetic tests must be translated into clinically relevant tools that can be readily incorporated into routine practice. Standardization of testing protocols, interpretation guidelines, and

integration with existing diagnostic algorithms is essential for widespread adoption.
- **Ethical and Privacy Considerations:** Genetic testing raises important ethical and privacy considerations related to informed consent, data security, and potential psychosocial implications of genetic risk disclosure. Clinicians must adhere to ethical guidelines and provide appropriate counseling and support to patients undergoing genetic testing.

Conclusion:

Biomarkers and genetic testing hold promise for advancing our understanding and management of cluster headaches. By elucidating underlying pathophysiological mechanisms, identifying genetic predispositions, and guiding treatment decisions, these tools offer opportunities for personalized approaches to diagnosis and therapy. Continued research efforts, collaboration between multidisciplinary teams, and integration of biomarkers and genetic testing into clinical practice are essential for improving outcomes and quality of life for individuals affected by cluster headaches.

CHAPTER 5: ACUTE AND PREVENTIVE TREATMENT APPROACHES

Pharmacological Interventions: Acute Relief

Pharmacological interventions play a central role in the management of cluster headaches, providing acute relief from the excruciating pain and associated symptoms characteristic of this disorder. Prompt and effective treatment is essential to alleviate the intensity and duration of cluster headache attacks, improve patient comfort, and minimize disability. This subchapter explores the pharmacological agents commonly used for acute relief in cluster headaches, highlighting their mechanisms of action, efficacy, and clinical considerations.

1. Oxygen Therapy:

- **Mechanism of Action:** Oxygen therapy is a cornerstone of acute relief for cluster headaches, exerting its effects by rapidly increasing arterial oxygen tension and alleviating hypoxia-induced cerebral vasodilation. Inhalation of 100% oxygen at a flow rate of 7-12 liters per minute for

15-20 minutes is typically employed during acute attacks.
- **Efficacy:** Oxygen therapy is highly effective in aborting cluster headache attacks, with response rates ranging from 70% to 80% in clinical studies. The onset of relief is rapid, typically within 15 minutes of initiating treatment, making it an ideal first-line intervention for acute management.
- **Clinical Considerations:** Oxygen therapy is safe, well-tolerated, and devoid of significant adverse effects when administered as directed. It can be self-administered by patients at home using portable oxygen cylinders or concentrators, providing convenient access to acute relief.

2. Triptans:

- **Mechanism of Action:** Triptans, serotonin receptor agonists, exert their therapeutic effects by activating serotonin (5-HT1B/1D) receptors and inhibiting the release of vasoactive neuropeptides involved in pain transmission and inflammation. Subcutaneous sumatriptan is the most commonly used triptan formulation for acute relief in cluster headaches.
- **Efficacy:** Triptans are effective in aborting cluster headache attacks, with response rates ranging from 60% to 80% in clinical trials. Subcutaneous sumatriptan is particularly fast-acting, with onset of relief within 10-15 minutes, making it a valuable option for patients requiring rapid pain relief.
- **Clinical Considerations:** Triptans are generally well-tolerated, but side effects such as transient flushing, chest tightness, or injection site reactions may occur. Contraindications, including coronary artery disease, uncontrolled hypertension, and use of monoamine oxidase inhibitors (MAOIs), should be considered before initiating treatment.

3. Intranasal Lidocaine:

- **Mechanism of Action:** Intranasal lidocaine acts as a local anesthetic, inhibiting nociceptive transmission along the trigeminal nerve fibers and modulating pain processing within the trigeminal autonomic reflex pathway. It is administered as a spray into the affected nostril during acute cluster headache attacks.
- **Efficacy:** Intranasal lidocaine has demonstrated efficacy in providing rapid relief from cluster headache pain, with response rates ranging from 60% to 70% in clinical studies. Onset of action is typically within 5-10 minutes, making it a useful adjunctive therapy for patients with contraindications to or inadequate response to other acute treatments.
- **Clinical Considerations:** Intranasal lidocaine is generally well-tolerated, but transient nasal discomfort or irritation may occur following administration. Caution is advised in patients with a history of sensitivity to local anesthetics or mucosal trauma.

4. Non-Steroidal Anti-Inflammatory Drugs (NSAIDs):

- **Mechanism of Action:** NSAIDs exert their analgesic and anti-inflammatory effects by inhibiting cyclooxygenase (COX) enzymes and reducing the synthesis of prostaglandins involved in pain and inflammation. Oral NSAIDs, such as ibuprofen or naproxen, are commonly used for acute relief in milder cluster headache attacks.
- **Efficacy:** NSAIDs may provide modest relief from cluster headache pain, particularly in less severe attacks or as adjunctive therapy to other acute treatments. However, their efficacy in aborting attacks is variable, and they are generally considered less effective than oxygen therapy or triptans.

- **Clinical Considerations:** NSAIDs are generally well-tolerated, but gastrointestinal irritation, renal impairment, and cardiovascular risks may limit their long-term use. Caution is advised in patients with a history of peptic ulcer disease, renal insufficiency, or cardiovascular disease.

5. **Corticosteroids:**

    - **Mechanism of Action:** Corticosteroids exert anti-inflammatory and immunomodulatory effects by inhibiting cytokine production, leukocyte migration, and prostaglandin synthesis. Intravenous or oral corticosteroids, such as prednisone or dexamethasone, may be used for short-term acute relief in cluster headaches.
    - **Efficacy:** Corticosteroids are effective in rapidly aborting cluster headache attacks and preventing recurrence during cluster periods. They are particularly useful as bridge therapy while initiating preventive treatments or during transitions between episodic and chronic cluster headache states.
    - **Clinical Considerations:** Corticosteroids are associated with potential adverse effects, including hyperglycemia, gastrointestinal bleeding, immunosuppression, and mood disturbances. Short-term use at the lowest effective dose is recommended to minimize risks.

Conclusion: Pharmacological interventions for acute relief play a vital role in the management of cluster headaches, providing rapid and effective relief from debilitating pain and associated symptoms. Oxygen therapy, triptans, intranasal lidocaine, NSAIDs, and corticosteroids are among the mainstays of acute treatment, each offering unique mechanisms of action, efficacy profiles, and clinical considerations. Individualized treatment strategies, based on the severity and frequency of attacks, patient preferences, and comorbidities, are essential for optimizing acute management and improving outcomes for patients with cluster headaches.

Pharmacological Interventions: Preventive Strategies

In addition to acute relief, pharmacological interventions are also employed for preventive management of cluster headaches. Preventive therapies aim to reduce the frequency, severity, and duration of cluster periods, thereby improving patients' quality of life and minimizing disability. This subchapter explores the pharmacological agents commonly used for preventive strategies in cluster headaches, their mechanisms of action, efficacy, and clinical considerations.

1. Verapamil:

- **Mechanism of Action**: Verapamil, a calcium channel blocker, is the cornerstone of preventive therapy for cluster headaches. It exerts its therapeutic effects by inhibiting calcium influx into vascular smooth muscle cells, reducing vasodilation, and modulating neurotransmitter release within the trigeminal-autonomic reflex pathway.
- **Efficacy:** Verapamil has demonstrated efficacy in reducing the frequency and severity of cluster headache attacks, with response rates ranging from 70% to 80% in clinical studies. It is considered the first-line preventive treatment for cluster headaches due to its proven efficacy and favorable side effect profile.
- **Clinical Considerations:** Verapamil should be initiated at a low dose and titrated gradually to achieve therapeutic response while minimizing adverse effects, such as hypotension, bradycardia, constipation, and peripheral edema. Close monitoring of blood pressure, heart rate,

and electrocardiogram (ECG) is recommended during dose escalation.

2. Lithium:

- **Mechanism of Action:** Lithium, a mood stabilizer, is commonly used for preventive therapy in cluster headaches, although its precise mechanism of action remains unclear. It may modulate neurotransmitter systems, including serotonin and glutamate, and exert anti-inflammatory effects that contribute to its therapeutic efficacy.
- **Efficacy:** Lithium has demonstrated efficacy in reducing the frequency and severity of cluster headache attacks, particularly in chronic cluster headache patients. Response rates vary, with approximately 50% of patients experiencing significant improvement in symptoms. Lithium is often reserved for patients who do not respond to or tolerate other preventive treatments.
- **Clinical Considerations:** Lithium requires regular monitoring of serum levels to ensure therapeutic efficacy and minimize toxicity. Common side effects include polyuria, polydipsia, tremor, weight gain, and gastrointestinal disturbances. Renal and thyroid function should be monitored regularly due to the potential for adverse effects on these organ systems.

3. Topiramate:

- **Mechanism of Action:** Topiramate, an antiepileptic drug, is occasionally used for preventive therapy in cluster headaches. Its mechanism of action involves modulation of voltage-gated ion channels, enhancement of gamma-aminobutyric acid (GABA) activity, and inhibition of glutamate-mediated excitatory neurotransmission.
- **Efficacy:** Topiramate has shown variable efficacy in

reducing the frequency and severity of cluster headache attacks, with response rates ranging from 30% to 50% in clinical studies. It may be considered as an alternative or adjunctive treatment in patients who do not respond to or tolerate other preventive therapies.

- **Clinical Considerations:** Topiramate is associated with a range of adverse effects, including cognitive impairment, weight loss, paresthesia, and metabolic disturbances. Dosing should be initiated at a low dose and titrated gradually to minimize side effects. Regular monitoring of cognitive function, electrolytes, and renal function is recommended during treatment.

4. Corticosteroids:

- **Mechanism of Action:** Corticosteroids, such as prednisone or dexamethasone, are occasionally used for short-term preventive therapy in cluster headaches. Their anti-inflammatory and immunomodulatory effects may help suppress neuroinflammatory processes and disrupt the neurovascular mechanisms underlying cluster headache pathogenesis.
- **Efficacy:** Corticosteroids are effective in rapidly attenuating cluster headache attacks and preventing recurrence during cluster periods. They are often used as bridge therapy while initiating long-term preventive treatments or during transitions between episodic and chronic cluster headache states.
- **Clinical Considerations:** Corticosteroids should be used cautiously for short-term preventive therapy due to the risk of adverse effects associated with long-term use, including hyperglycemia, hypertension, immunosuppression, and mood disturbances. Short courses at the lowest effective dose are recommended to minimize risks.

Conclusion: Pharmacological interventions for preventive management play a crucial role in reducing the burden of cluster headaches and improving patients' quality of life. Verapamil remains the first-line preventive treatment due to its proven efficacy and safety profile. Lithium, topiramate, and corticosteroids are considered alternative options for patients who do not respond to or tolerate verapamil or for those with specific clinical indications. Individualized treatment approaches, based on the severity and frequency of attacks, comorbidities, and patient preferences, are essential for

Non-Pharmacological Therapies: Neuromodulation Techniques

Non-pharmacological therapies, particularly neuromodulation techniques, have gained increasing recognition as adjunctive treatments for cluster headaches. These modalities offer alternative approaches to managing cluster headaches, especially in patients who are refractory to or intolerant of pharmacological interventions. This subchapter explores the various neuromodulation techniques employed in the management of cluster headaches, including their mechanisms of action, efficacy, and clinical considerations.

1. Occipital Nerve Stimulation (ONS):

- **Mechanism of Action:** Occipital nerve stimulation involves the percutaneous implantation of electrodes near the occipital nerves, with electrical impulses delivered to modulate pain transmission along the trigeminal and occipital nerve pathways. ONS is thought to exert its therapeutic effects by disrupting nociceptive signaling and inhibiting central sensitization mechanisms.
- **Efficacy:** ONS has demonstrated efficacy in reducing the frequency, intensity, and duration of cluster headache

attacks, with response rates ranging from 50% to 70% in clinical studies. It is particularly effective in patients with refractory chronic cluster headaches who have failed to respond to other treatments.
- **Clinical Considerations:** ONS implantation is performed as a surgical procedure under local anesthesia, requiring careful patient selection, electrode placement, and programming of stimulation parameters. Adverse effects may include lead migration, infection, hardware malfunction, and discomfort at the implant site.

2. Transcutaneous Supraorbital Nerve Stimulation (tSNS):

- **Mechanism of Action:** Transcutaneous supraorbital nerve stimulation involves the application of electrical impulses to the supraorbital nerves using external electrodes placed on the forehead. tSNS modulates pain processing within the trigeminal nerve pathway and trigeminal autonomic reflex, potentially interrupting the development of cluster headache attacks.
- **Efficacy:** tSNS has demonstrated efficacy in reducing the frequency and intensity of cluster headache attacks, with response rates ranging from 50% to 60% in clinical studies. It is well-tolerated and may offer a non-invasive alternative for patients who prefer or cannot undergo invasive procedures.
- **Clinical Considerations:** tSNS devices are portable and can be self-administered by patients at home during cluster headache attacks. Optimal electrode placement, stimulation parameters, and treatment duration should be determined based on individual response and tolerability.

3. Deep Brain Stimulation (DBS):

- **Mechanism of Action:** Deep brain stimulation involves the implantation of electrodes within specific deep

brain structures implicated in pain processing, such as the hypothalamus or periaqueductal gray matter. DBS modulates neural activity and neurotransmitter release within these regions, potentially disrupting abnormal pain circuitry associated with cluster headaches.
- **Efficacy:** DBS has shown promising results in reducing the frequency and severity of cluster headache attacks, particularly in patients with refractory chronic cluster headaches. Response rates vary, with approximately 50% to 70% of patients experiencing significant improvement in symptoms.
- **Clinical Considerations:** DBS is an invasive surgical procedure that requires precise targeting of electrode placement and careful programming of stimulation parameters. Adverse effects may include lead migration, infection, hardware malfunction, and neuropsychiatric symptoms.

4. Vagus Nerve Stimulation (VNS):

- **Mechanism of Action:** Vagus nerve stimulation involves the implantation of a device that delivers electrical impulses to the cervical vagus nerve, modulating central and peripheral pathways involved in pain modulation and autonomic regulation. VNS may exert anti-inflammatory, neuromodulatory, and neuroprotective effects relevant to cluster headache pathophysiology.
- **Efficacy:** VNS has shown promising results in reducing the frequency and severity of cluster headache attacks, although evidence remains limited compared to other neuromodulation techniques. Response rates vary, with some patients experiencing significant improvement in symptoms.
- **Clinical Considerations:** VNS implantation is an invasive procedure requiring careful patient selection, electrode placement, and programming of stimulation parameters.

Adverse effects may include voice alteration, coughing, neck pain, and infection at the implant site.

Conclusion: Neuromodulation techniques offer alternative approaches to managing cluster headaches, particularly in patients who do not respond to or tolerate pharmacological interventions. Occipital nerve stimulation, transcutaneous supraorbital nerve stimulation, deep brain stimulation, and vagus nerve stimulation have shown promise in reducing the frequency, intensity, and duration of cluster headache attacks, although further research is needed to elucidate their mechanisms of action and optimize treatment protocols. Individualized approaches, based on patient preferences, treatment responsiveness, and clinical considerations, are essential for selecting appropriate neuromodulation therapies and maximizing outcomes for patients with cluster headaches.

Surgical and Invasive Procedures

Surgical and invasive procedures represent additional therapeutic options for patients with cluster headaches, particularly those who are refractory to standard pharmacological and non-pharmacological treatments. These interventions aim to modulate pain pathways, interrupt nociceptive signaling, and provide long-term relief from cluster headache symptoms. This subchapter explores various surgical and invasive procedures employed in the management of cluster headaches, including their indications, techniques, efficacy, and clinical considerations.

1. Microvascular Decompression (MVD):

- **Indications:** Microvascular decompression involves surgical exploration and decompression of the trigeminal nerve root entry zone to alleviate compression by vascular structures, such as the superior cerebellar artery or cranial nerve VII. MVD may be considered in patients with refractory cluster headaches and evidence of neurovascular compression on imaging studies.

- **Technique:** During MVD, a small craniotomy is performed to expose the trigeminal nerve root entry zone, and vascular compressions are identified and decompressed using Teflon pledgets or similar materials. The goal is to relieve mechanical irritation of the trigeminal nerve and disrupt aberrant pain signaling pathways.
- **Efficacy:** MVD has shown variable efficacy in reducing the frequency and severity of cluster headache attacks in select patients with neurovascular compression syndromes. Response rates range from 50% to 70%, with some patients experiencing long-term remission of symptoms.
- **Clinical Considerations:** MVD is a complex surgical procedure associated with risks of intracranial hemorrhage, cerebrospinal fluid leak, facial nerve injury, and hearing loss. Careful patient selection, meticulous surgical technique, and postoperative monitoring are essential for optimizing outcomes.

2. Glycerol Rhizotomy:

- **Indications:** Glycerol rhizotomy involves percutaneous injection of glycerol into the trigeminal cistern to disrupt trigeminal nerve function and alleviate pain. It may be considered in patients with refractory cluster headaches who have failed to respond to pharmacological and non-pharmacological treatments.
- **Technique:** Glycerol rhizotomy is performed under fluoroscopic guidance, with a needle inserted into the trigeminal cistern via a percutaneous approach. Glycerol is injected to induce chemical ablation of the trigeminal nerve fibers, thereby interrupting pain transmission.
- **Efficacy:** Glycerol rhizotomy has shown variable efficacy

in providing long-term relief from cluster headache symptoms, with response rates ranging from 50% to 70%. The duration of pain relief may vary, with some patients experiencing prolonged remission of symptoms.
- **Clinical Considerations:** Glycerol rhizotomy carries risks of facial numbness, corneal anesthesia, dysesthesias, and cerebrospinal fluid leakage. Patient selection, procedural technique, and post-procedural monitoring are critical for minimizing complications and optimizing outcomes.

3. Radiofrequency Thermocoagulation:

- **Indications:** Radiofrequency thermocoagulation involves percutaneous application of heat energy to the trigeminal nerve branches to disrupt nociceptive signaling and provide pain relief. It may be considered in patients with refractory cluster headaches who have not responded to other treatments.
- **Technique:** Radiofrequency thermocoagulation is performed under fluoroscopic guidance, with a radiofrequency electrode inserted percutaneously to target the trigeminal nerve branches responsible for cluster headache pain. Heat energy is then delivered to create thermal lesions, interrupting pain transmission.
- **Efficacy:** Radiofrequency thermocoagulation has shown variable efficacy in reducing the frequency and intensity of cluster headache attacks, with response rates ranging from 50% to 70%. The duration of pain relief may vary, and repeat procedures may be necessary to maintain efficacy.
- **Clinical Considerations:** Radiofrequency thermocoagulation carries risks of facial numbness, dysesthesias, corneal anesthesia, and motor deficits. Careful patient selection, procedural technique, and post-procedural monitoring are essential for minimizing complications and optimizing outcomes.

4. Deep Brain Stimulation (DBS):

- **Indications:** Deep brain stimulation involves the implantation of electrodes within specific deep brain structures implicated in pain processing, such as the hypothalamus or periaqueductal gray matter. DBS may be considered in patients with refractory chronic cluster headaches who have failed to respond to other treatments.
- **Technique:** DBS implantation involves stereotactic neurosurgical techniques to precisely target electrode placement within the deep brain structures implicated in cluster headache pathophysiology. Electrical impulses are then delivered via an implanted pulse generator to modulate neural activity and disrupt abnormal pain circuitry.
- **Efficacy:** DBS has shown promising results in reducing the frequency and severity of cluster headache attacks, with response rates ranging from 50% to 70% in clinical studies. Long-term follow-up data suggest sustained efficacy and improvements in quality of life for some patients.
- **Clinical Considerations:** DBS is an invasive surgical procedure associated with risks of intracranial hemorrhage, infection, hardware malfunction, and neuropsychiatric symptoms. Careful patient selection, electrode targeting, programming, and postoperative management are essential for optimizing outcomes.

Conclusion: Surgical and invasive procedures offer additional therapeutic options for patients with refractory cluster headaches who have not responded to standard pharmacological and non-pharmacological treatments. Microvascular decompression, glycerol rhizotomy, radiofrequency thermocoagulation, and deep brain stimulation are among the surgical interventions employed to modulate pain pathways, interrupt nociceptive signaling, and provide long-term relief from cluster headache symptoms. Careful patient selection, procedural technique, and post-procedural monitoring are essential for optimizing outcomes and minimizing complications.

Combination Therapies and Emerging Treatments

Combination therapies and emerging treatments represent innovative approaches in the management of cluster headaches, offering potential synergistic effects, improved efficacy, and novel mechanisms of action. This subchapter explores the concept of combining multiple treatment modalities and highlights emerging therapeutic strategies that hold promise for enhancing outcomes in patients with cluster headaches.

1. Combination Therapies:

- **Rationale:** Combination therapies involve the simultaneous or sequential use of multiple pharmacological and non-pharmacological interventions to target different aspects of cluster headache pathophysiology and provide synergistic relief. Combining treatments with complementary mechanisms of action may enhance efficacy, reduce the frequency of attacks, and improve overall symptom control.
- **Examples:** Common combination therapies for cluster headaches include the concurrent use of verapamil with a subcutaneous triptan for acute relief, or the combination of occipital nerve stimulation with preventive medications such as lithium or topiramate. Non-pharmacological interventions, such as lifestyle modifications, stress management techniques, and behavioral therapies, may also be integrated into comprehensive treatment plans.
- **Clinical Considerations:** Combination therapies should be

individualized based on the patient's clinical presentation, treatment responsiveness, tolerability, and preferences. Close monitoring of treatment response, adverse effects, and potential drug interactions is essential to optimize therapeutic outcomes and minimize risks.

2. Emerging Treatments:

- **Novel Pharmacological Agents:** Several novel pharmacological agents are under investigation for the treatment of cluster headaches, targeting specific neurochemical pathways implicated in the disorder. These include calcitonin gene-related peptide (CGRP) receptor antagonists, pituitary adenylate cyclase-activating polypeptide (PACAP) receptor antagonists, and glutamate receptor modulators. Early clinical trials have shown promising results in reducing the frequency and severity of cluster headache attacks, with fewer adverse effects compared to traditional treatments.
- **Neuromodulation Technologies:** Advancements in neuromodulation technologies continue to expand the therapeutic options for cluster headaches. Novel approaches, such as sphenopalatine ganglion stimulation, transcranial magnetic stimulation, and non-invasive vagus nerve stimulation, are being investigated for their potential to modulate pain pathways, disrupt trigeminal autonomic reflexes, and provide sustained relief from cluster headache symptoms.
- **Gene Therapy:** Gene therapy holds promise as a targeted approach to modulate gene expression, neurochemical signaling, and neuroinflammatory processes implicated in cluster headache pathogenesis. Preclinical studies have explored the use of viral vectors to deliver therapeutic genes encoding anti-inflammatory cytokines, neuropeptides, or neurotransmitter receptors to specific brain regions involved in pain processing. Clinical trials

are underway to evaluate the safety and efficacy of gene therapy approaches in patients with refractory cluster headaches.

Conclusion: Combination therapies and emerging treatments offer exciting opportunities to improve outcomes and quality of life for patients with cluster headaches. By combining multiple treatment modalities with complementary mechanisms of action and exploring novel therapeutic strategies targeting specific pathophysiological pathways, clinicians can tailor treatment plans to individual patient needs, optimize symptom control, and minimize disability. Further research and clinical trials are needed to validate the efficacy, safety, and long-term outcomes of these innovative approaches and expand the armamentarium of treatments available for cluster headaches.

CHAPTER 6: LIFESTYLE MODIFICATIONS AND HOLISTIC MANAGEMENT

Importance of Sleep Hygiene and Stress Management

Effective management of cluster headaches extends beyond pharmacological and procedural interventions to encompass lifestyle modifications and psychosocial strategies. Sleep hygiene and stress management play pivotal roles in the prevention and mitigation of cluster headache attacks. This subchapter explores the importance of sleep hygiene and stress management techniques in the management of cluster headaches, highlighting their impact on disease course, symptom severity, and overall quality of life.

1. Sleep Hygiene:

- **Definition:** Sleep hygiene refers to a set of behavioral and environmental practices that promote healthy sleep patterns and optimize sleep quality. Good sleep hygiene habits are essential for regulating circadian rhythms, promoting restorative sleep, and minimizing triggers for

cluster headache attacks.
- **Key Practices:** Important aspects of sleep hygiene include maintaining a consistent sleep schedule, creating a comfortable sleep environment (e.g., dark, quiet, and cool), avoiding stimulating activities before bedtime, limiting exposure to screens and electronic devices, and practicing relaxation techniques to facilitate sleep onset.
- **Impact on Cluster Headaches:** Disruptions in sleep patterns, such as irregular sleep schedules, poor sleep quality, and sleep deprivation, have been linked to an increased risk of cluster headache attacks and exacerbation of symptoms. Improving sleep hygiene practices may help stabilize circadian rhythms, reduce the frequency and intensity of attacks, and enhance treatment responsiveness.

2. Stress Management:

- **Definition:** Stress management encompasses a variety of techniques aimed at reducing psychological and physiological stress responses, promoting relaxation, and enhancing coping mechanisms. Chronic stress and emotional distress are common triggers for cluster headache attacks and can exacerbate symptom severity.
- **Techniques:** Effective stress management techniques include mindfulness meditation, deep breathing exercises, progressive muscle relaxation, biofeedback, cognitive-behavioral therapy (CBT), and stress-reducing activities such as yoga, tai chi, and massage therapy. These approaches help alleviate muscle tension, regulate autonomic function, and modulate pain perception pathways.
- **Impact on Cluster Headaches:** Stressful life events, emotional upheavals, and maladaptive coping strategies have been implicated in the onset and exacerbation of cluster headache attacks. By incorporating stress

management techniques into daily routines, individuals with cluster headaches can better cope with triggers, reduce the frequency and intensity of attacks, and improve overall well-being.

3. Holistic Approach:

- **Integration with Treatment:** Sleep hygiene and stress management techniques should be integrated into comprehensive treatment plans for cluster headaches, alongside pharmacological, non-pharmacological, and interventional strategies. A holistic approach addresses the multifactorial nature of cluster headaches and empowers patients to actively participate in their own care.
- **Patient Education:** Educating patients about the importance of sleep hygiene and stress management is crucial for fostering self-awareness, promoting adherence to healthy behaviors, and empowering individuals to identify and mitigate triggers for cluster headache attacks. Clinicians should provide guidance on implementing practical strategies and overcoming barriers to behavior change.
- **Multidisciplinary Collaboration:** Collaboration between healthcare providers, including neurologists, primary care physicians, psychologists, and sleep specialists, is essential for delivering comprehensive care and addressing the complex interplay between sleep, stress, and cluster headaches. Multidisciplinary approaches facilitate individualized treatment plans tailored to each patient's needs and preferences.

Conclusion: Sleep hygiene and stress management are integral components of cluster headache management, offering complementary approaches to pharmacological and procedural interventions. By promoting healthy sleep patterns, reducing stress levels, and enhancing coping mechanisms, individuals with cluster headaches can optimize symptom control, minimize trigger exposure, and improve overall quality of life. Incorporating sleep hygiene and stress management techniques into comprehensive treatment plans requires a holistic approach, patient education, and multidisciplinary collaboration to address the multifactorial nature of cluster headaches and promote long-term wellness.

Dietary Considerations and Trigger Avoidance

Dietary considerations and trigger avoidance strategies are essential components of the management plan for individuals with cluster headaches. Certain foods, beverages, and dietary habits have been identified as potential triggers for cluster headache attacks, and making informed dietary choices can help reduce the frequency and severity of episodes. This subchapter explores the role of dietary factors in cluster headaches and provides guidance on trigger avoidance strategies.

1. Identifying Dietary Triggers:

- **Common Triggers:** Certain foods and beverages have been reported to trigger cluster headache attacks in susceptible individuals. Common dietary triggers include alcohol (especially red wine), aged cheeses, cured meats (such as bacon and salami), chocolate, caffeine, monosodium glutamate (MSG), and artificial sweeteners (such as aspartame).
- **Individual Variability:** Triggers can vary widely among individuals, and not all individuals with cluster headaches are sensitive to the same dietary factors. Keeping a detailed headache diary can help identify personal triggers by tracking food and beverage consumption alongside headache occurrence.

2. Implementing Trigger Avoidance:

- **Elimination Diet:** For individuals who suspect specific dietary triggers, an elimination diet may be recommended under the guidance of a healthcare professional or registered dietitian. This involves temporarily removing potential trigger foods from the diet and gradually reintroducing them one at a time while monitoring for headache occurrence.
- **Healthy Dietary Habits:** In addition to avoiding specific triggers, adopting a well-balanced and nutritious diet can help support overall health and potentially reduce the frequency and severity of cluster headache attacks. Emphasizing whole foods such as fruits, vegetables, lean proteins, whole grains, and healthy fats while minimizing processed and high-fat foods may be beneficial.

3. Hydration and Fluid Intake:

- **Dehydration:** Dehydration can exacerbate headache symptoms and trigger cluster headache attacks in susceptible individuals. Maintaining adequate hydration by drinking plenty of water throughout the day is important for preventing dehydration-related headaches.
- **Avoiding Triggers:** Certain beverages, such as alcohol and caffeinated beverages, can act as triggers for cluster headaches in some individuals. Limiting or avoiding these beverages, especially during cluster periods or when experiencing prodromal symptoms, may help reduce the risk of headache onset.

4. Individualized Approach:

- **Personalized Recommendations:** Due to the individual variability in triggers and responses, dietary recommendations should be personalized based on

each individual's experience and sensitivities. Healthcare providers can work collaboratively with patients to identify triggers, develop tailored dietary plans, and provide guidance on making sustainable lifestyle changes.
- **Patient Education:** Educating patients about the potential impact of diet on cluster headaches and empowering them to make informed dietary choices is essential for successful management. Providing resources, such as lists of common triggers and practical tips for avoiding triggers, can support patients in implementing dietary modifications.

Conclusion: Dietary considerations and trigger avoidance strategies play a significant role in the management of cluster headaches. By identifying and avoiding potential dietary triggers, individuals with cluster headaches can potentially reduce the frequency and severity of attacks. Adopting healthy dietary habits, staying hydrated, and working with healthcare providers to develop personalized dietary plans are important steps towards optimizing symptom control and improving quality of life for individuals living with cluster headaches.

Physical Activity and Exercise Recommendations

Physical activity and exercise are important components of a comprehensive management plan for individuals with cluster headaches. While the relationship between exercise and cluster headaches is complex and can vary among individuals, regular physical activity has been associated with numerous health benefits, including improved mood, stress reduction, and enhanced overall well-being. This subchapter explores the role of physical activity and exercise in the management of cluster headaches and provides recommendations for incorporating exercise into daily routines.

1. **Benefits of Physical Activity:**

    - **Mood Enhancement:** Regular physical activity has been shown to release endorphins, serotonin, and other neurotransmitters that contribute to mood improvement and stress reduction. Engaging in exercise can help alleviate symptoms of anxiety and depression commonly associated with cluster headaches.
    - **Stress Reduction:** Physical activity serves as a natural stress reliever, helping to reduce tension, promote relaxation, and improve coping mechanisms. Managing stress levels is important for minimizing triggers and preventing exacerbation of cluster headache attacks.
    - **Improved Overall Health:** Regular exercise contributes to cardiovascular health, weight management, and overall physical fitness. Maintaining a healthy lifestyle through regular physical activity may help reduce the frequency and severity of cluster headache attacks and improve general well-being.

2. **Exercise Recommendations:**

    - **Moderate Intensity:** Engaging in moderate-intensity aerobic exercise, such as brisk walking, cycling, swimming, or jogging, for at least 150 minutes per week is recommended for overall health benefits. Incorporating strength training exercises, such as weightlifting or bodyweight exercises, two or more days per week can further enhance muscle strength and endurance.
    - **Gradual Progression:** Individuals with cluster headaches should start with low-impact exercises and gradually increase intensity and duration based on individual tolerance and symptom response. It is essential to listen to the body and avoid overexertion, particularly during cluster periods or when experiencing prodromal

symptoms.
- **Consistency:** Consistency is key to reaping the benefits of exercise. Establishing a regular exercise routine and incorporating physical activity into daily life, such as taking the stairs, walking or cycling for transportation, or participating in recreational activities, can help maintain momentum and adherence over the long term.

3. Considerations for Individuals with Cluster Headaches:

- **Timing:** Some individuals may find that engaging in exercise during a cluster headache attack exacerbates symptoms or triggers an attack. In such cases, it may be preferable to schedule exercise sessions during headache-free periods or when symptoms are less severe.
- **Hydration and Rest:** Staying hydrated and ensuring adequate rest and recovery are important considerations for individuals with cluster headaches engaging in physical activity. Proper hydration can help prevent dehydration-related headaches, while adequate rest allows the body to recover and minimize fatigue.
- **Individualized Approach:** Exercise recommendations should be tailored to each individual's preferences, capabilities, and medical history. Healthcare providers can provide guidance on appropriate exercise modalities, intensity levels, and safety precautions based on individual needs.

4. Incorporating Variety:**

- **Mixing it Up:** Incorporating a variety of physical activities and exercise modalities can help prevent boredom, enhance motivation, and target different muscle groups. Activities such as yoga, Pilates, tai chi, and recreational sports offer additional benefits, including flexibility, balance, and relaxation.

- **Adaptability:** Individuals with cluster headaches may experience fluctuations in symptoms and energy levels. Being adaptable and flexible with exercise routines, adjusting intensity or duration as needed, can help accommodate changes in symptom severity and ensure continued participation in physical activity.

Conclusion: Physical activity and exercise play a crucial role in the management of cluster headaches, offering numerous benefits for overall health and well-being. By incorporating regular exercise into daily routines, individuals with cluster headaches can experience mood enhancement, stress reduction, and improvements in physical fitness. Adhering to exercise recommendations, listening to the body, and adopting an individualized approach can help maximize the benefits of physical activity while minimizing the risk of exacerbating cluster headache symptoms.

Mindfulness, Meditation, and Relaxation Techniques

Mindfulness, meditation, and relaxation techniques are valuable tools in the management of cluster headaches, offering individuals effective strategies to cope with pain, reduce stress, and enhance overall well-being. These practices cultivate awareness, promote mental clarity, and foster a sense of calm, helping individuals navigate the challenges of living with cluster headaches. This subchapter explores the role of mindfulness, meditation, and relaxation techniques in cluster headache management and provides guidance on their implementation.

1. Mindfulness Practices:

- **Definition:** Mindfulness involves paying deliberate attention to the present moment, without judgment, and with an attitude of openness and acceptance. Mindfulness

practices cultivate awareness of thoughts, emotions, bodily sensations, and external stimuli, allowing individuals to respond to experiences with greater clarity and equanimity.
- **Benefits:** Mindfulness practices have been shown to reduce stress, alleviate symptoms of anxiety and depression, enhance pain tolerance, and improve overall quality of life. By fostering non-reactivity and acceptance, mindfulness can help individuals with cluster headaches navigate pain episodes with greater resilience and self-compassion.

2. Meditation Techniques:

- **Types of Meditation:** Various meditation techniques can be beneficial for individuals with cluster headaches, including focused attention meditation (e.g., mindful breathing, body scan), loving-kindness meditation (cultivating compassion and empathy), and mindfulness-based stress reduction (MBSR) practices. Each technique offers unique benefits and can be tailored to individual preferences and needs.
- **Mechanisms of Action:** Meditation practices promote relaxation, regulate autonomic nervous system function, modulate pain perception pathways, and enhance emotional regulation. Regular meditation practice can help individuals develop skills for self-regulation and coping with pain and stress.

3. Relaxation Techniques:

- **Progressive Muscle Relaxation:** Progressive muscle relaxation involves systematically tensing and releasing muscle groups throughout the body, promoting physical relaxation and reducing muscle tension. This technique can help alleviate symptoms of tension headaches and promote overall relaxation.

- **Deep Breathing Exercises:** Deep breathing exercises, such as diaphragmatic breathing or paced breathing, involve slow, rhythmic breathing patterns that activate the parasympathetic nervous system, induce relaxation, and reduce physiological arousal. Deep breathing can be practiced as a standalone technique or incorporated into mindfulness and meditation practices.

4. Integration into Daily Life:

- **Consistent Practice:** Consistency is key to reaping the benefits of mindfulness, meditation, and relaxation techniques. Establishing a regular practice routine, even if for brief periods each day, can help individuals build resilience, enhance coping skills, and maintain emotional balance amidst the challenges of living with cluster headaches.
- **Incorporating Informal Practices:** In addition to formal meditation sessions, individuals can integrate mindfulness and relaxation practices into daily activities, such as mindful eating, mindful walking, or taking short relaxation breaks throughout the day. Cultivating present-moment awareness in everyday life fosters a sense of groundedness and connection to the present moment.

5. Resources and Support:

- **Guided Practices:** Guided mindfulness and meditation practices, available through audio recordings, smartphone apps, or online platforms, can provide structured guidance and support for individuals new to these techniques. Guided sessions offer step-by-step instructions and prompts to help individuals navigate the practice effectively.
- **Community and Group Support:** Joining mindfulness or

meditation groups, participating in workshops or classes, or seeking guidance from qualified instructors or mental health professionals can provide additional support and accountability in establishing and maintaining a mindfulness practice.

Conclusion: Mindfulness, meditation, and relaxation techniques offer valuable tools for individuals with cluster headaches to manage pain, reduce stress, and enhance overall well-being. By cultivating present-moment awareness, developing emotional regulation skills, and fostering relaxation responses, individuals can navigate the challenges of living with cluster headaches with greater resilience and equanimity. Consistent practice, integration into daily life, and access to resources and support networks are essential for maximizing the benefits of these techniques and promoting holistic wellness.

Integrative Medicine Approaches: Acupuncture, Yoga, etc.

Integrative medicine approaches, such as acupuncture, yoga, and other complementary therapies, offer additional options for individuals seeking holistic management of cluster headaches. These modalities aim to restore balance, promote relaxation, and alleviate symptoms through non-pharmacological means. This subchapter explores the role of integrative medicine approaches in cluster headache management and provides insights into their potential benefits and considerations.

1. Acupuncture:

- **Principle:** Acupuncture is an ancient Chinese healing practice that involves the insertion of thin needles into specific points on the body to stimulate nerve-rich areas and promote natural healing processes. Traditional Chinese medicine theory suggests that acupuncture

rebalances the flow of vital energy, or Qi, along meridian pathways to alleviate pain and restore health.
- **Potential Benefits:** Acupuncture has been reported to provide relief from cluster headache symptoms, including pain intensity, frequency, and duration. Research suggests that acupuncture may modulate pain perception pathways, regulate neuroendocrine function, and reduce inflammation, contributing to its therapeutic effects.
- **Considerations:** While acupuncture is generally considered safe when performed by trained practitioners using sterile needles, individual responses may vary. Acupuncture may not be suitable for everyone, and it is important to discuss potential risks and benefits with a qualified healthcare provider before undergoing treatment.

2. Yoga:

- **Philosophy:** Yoga is a mind-body practice that originated in ancient India, incorporating physical postures, breathwork, meditation, and relaxation techniques to promote physical, mental, and spiritual well-being. Yoga philosophy emphasizes the interconnectedness of body, mind, and spirit and seeks to cultivate harmony and balance within the individual.
- **Potential Benefits:** Yoga has been shown to reduce stress, improve mood, enhance flexibility and strength, and promote relaxation, all of which may benefit individuals with cluster headaches. Certain yoga poses, breathing exercises (pranayama), and meditation techniques can help alleviate muscle tension, regulate autonomic function, and reduce stress-related triggers.
- **Adaptability:** Yoga practices can be adapted to accommodate individuals with varying abilities and health conditions. Gentle yoga styles, such as Hatha or Restorative yoga, may be particularly suitable for

individuals with cluster headaches, offering gentle movements, supportive props, and guided relaxation.

3. Mind-Body Medicine:

- **Biofeedback:** Biofeedback techniques involve monitoring and regulating physiological responses, such as heart rate, muscle tension, and skin temperature, using electronic monitoring devices. Biofeedback training teaches individuals to gain voluntary control over autonomic functions and reduce stress-related symptoms, potentially benefiting those with cluster headaches.
- **Tai Chi:** Tai Chi is a gentle form of Chinese martial arts that emphasizes slow, flowing movements, deep breathing, and mindfulness. Tai Chi practice promotes relaxation, balance, and coordination, while also improving muscle strength and flexibility. Preliminary research suggests that Tai Chi may help reduce headache frequency and improve quality of life in individuals with cluster headaches.

4. Herbal Medicine and Nutritional Supplements:

- **Herbal Remedies:** Certain herbal remedies, such as feverfew, butterbur, and riboflavin (vitamin B2), have been studied for their potential efficacy in preventing migraines and other types of headaches. While evidence specific to cluster headaches is limited, some individuals may find herbal remedies helpful as part of a comprehensive treatment approach. It is important to consult with a healthcare provider before using herbal supplements, as they may interact with medications or have contraindications.
- **Nutritional Supplements:** Certain nutritional supplements, such as magnesium, coenzyme Q10, and melatonin, have been investigated for their potential role in migraine and headache management. While research

on their efficacy in cluster headaches is ongoing, some individuals may benefit from supplementation under the guidance of a qualified healthcare provider.

Conclusion: Integrative medicine approaches, including acupuncture, yoga, mind-body practices, and herbal medicine, offer additional options for individuals seeking holistic management of cluster headaches. These modalities complement conventional treatments by addressing underlying imbalances, promoting relaxation, and enhancing overall well-being. While integrative approaches may not be suitable for everyone, they can provide valuable tools for individuals seeking to optimize symptom control, reduce medication reliance, and improve quality of life. Collaboration between healthcare providers and individuals with cluster headaches is essential for developing personalized treatment plans that incorporate both conventional and integrative modalities to meet individual needs

CHAPTER 7: COMORBIDITIES AND PSYCHOSOCIAL IMPACT

Associated Conditions: Depression, Anxiety, Sleep Disorders

Individuals with cluster headaches often experience comorbidities such as depression, anxiety, and sleep disorders, which can significantly impact their overall quality of life and exacerbate headache symptoms. Understanding and addressing these associated conditions are essential aspects of comprehensive cluster headache management. This subchapter explores the relationship between cluster headaches and associated conditions, their impact on disease course, and strategies for assessment and management.

1. Depression:

- **Prevalence:** Depression is common among individuals with cluster headaches, with studies reporting a higher prevalence compared to the general population. The chronic and disabling nature of cluster headaches, along

with the burden of frequent attacks, can contribute to feelings of hopelessness, despair, and low mood.
- **Impact:** Depression can exacerbate headache symptoms, impair cognitive function, and negatively affect treatment adherence and response. Individuals with cluster headaches and comorbid depression may experience greater disability, reduced quality of life, and increased healthcare utilization.
- **Assessment and Management:** Screening for depression should be incorporated into routine clinical assessments for individuals with cluster headaches. Treatment may involve a combination of pharmacotherapy, psychotherapy (such as cognitive-behavioral therapy), lifestyle modifications, and social support interventions. Collaboration between neurologists, primary care providers, and mental health professionals is essential for optimizing outcomes.

2. Anxiety:

- **Prevalence:** Anxiety disorders are common among individuals with cluster headaches, with symptoms ranging from generalized anxiety to panic attacks and phobias. The unpredictable nature of cluster headache attacks and the fear of experiencing severe pain can contribute to heightened anxiety levels.
- **Impact:** Anxiety can exacerbate headache frequency and severity, increase sensitivity to pain, and interfere with daily functioning. Individuals with cluster headaches and comorbid anxiety may experience greater distress, avoidance behaviors, and impairment in social and occupational domains.
- **Assessment and Management:** Screening for anxiety disorders should be included in comprehensive evaluations for individuals with cluster headaches. Treatment may involve pharmacotherapy (such as

anxiolytics or antidepressants), cognitive-behavioral therapy, relaxation techniques, and stress management strategies. Addressing anxiety symptoms can improve overall well-being and enhance coping with cluster headache attacks.

3. Sleep Disorders:

- **Prevalence:** Sleep disturbances are common in individuals with cluster headaches, with reports of insomnia, sleep fragmentation, and sleep-related breathing disorders. Cluster headache attacks, nocturnal onset of symptoms, and associated nocturnal awakenings can disrupt sleep architecture and lead to poor sleep quality.
- **Impact:** Sleep disorders can exacerbate cluster headache symptoms, trigger attacks, and contribute to daytime fatigue, cognitive impairment, and mood disturbances. Poor sleep quality may also impair treatment response and recovery from headache episodes.
- **Assessment and Management:** Evaluation of sleep patterns and sleep disorders should be integral to the assessment of individuals with cluster headaches. Treatment may involve sleep hygiene education, cognitive-behavioral therapy for insomnia (CBT-I), pharmacotherapy for sleep disorders (such as hypnotics or melatonin), and addressing underlying sleep-related breathing abnormalities. Improving sleep quality can help reduce headache frequency, enhance daytime functioning, and improve overall quality of life.

Conclusion: Associated conditions such as depression, anxiety, and sleep disorders are common among individuals with cluster headaches and can significantly impact disease course and overall well-being. Understanding the interplay between cluster headaches and comorbidities is essential for comprehensive management. Screening, assessment, and targeted interventions for depression, anxiety, and sleep disorders are integral components of holistic cluster headache care, aimed at optimizing treatment outcomes and improving quality of life for affected individuals. Collaborative efforts between healthcare providers across disciplines are essential for addressing the complex needs of individuals with cluster headaches and associated conditions.

Impact on Relationships and Social Functioning

Cluster headaches not only affect individuals physically but also have significant repercussions on their relationships and social functioning. The unpredictable nature and severity of cluster headache attacks can strain interpersonal relationships, disrupt social activities, and impede daily functioning. Understanding the impact of cluster headaches on relationships and social interactions is crucial for providing comprehensive care and support. This subchapter delves into the challenges faced by individuals with cluster headaches in maintaining relationships and participating in social activities, as well as strategies for coping and fostering support networks.

1. Strain on Relationships:

- **Communication Challenges:** Individuals with cluster headaches may find it difficult to communicate the severity and unpredictability of their symptoms to family members, friends, and colleagues. Misunderstandings about the nature of cluster headaches, frustration with treatment outcomes, and the burden of caregiving responsibilities can strain relationships.
- **Emotional Toll:** Cluster headaches can take a toll on the emotional well-being of both patients and their loved ones. Feelings of helplessness, guilt, resentment, and isolation may arise, leading to conflicts and emotional

distance within relationships. Partners, family members, and caregivers may experience stress and burnout from witnessing the suffering of their loved ones.

2. Social Isolation:

- **Avoidance of Social Activities:** Fear of experiencing cluster headache attacks in public settings or being unable to participate fully in social activities may lead individuals to avoid socializing altogether. The need to retreat to a quiet, dark environment during attacks can result in social withdrawal and feelings of loneliness and isolation.
- **Impact on Work and Social Roles:** Cluster headaches can disrupt occupational functioning and limit participation in social roles and responsibilities. Absences from work, decreased productivity, and difficulty maintaining social commitments may lead to feelings of inadequacy and loss of identity.

3. Coping Strategies:

- **Open Communication:** Open and honest communication between individuals with cluster headaches and their loved ones is essential for fostering understanding, empathy, and support. Sharing experiences, expressing needs and concerns, and setting realistic expectations can strengthen relationships and alleviate feelings of isolation.
- **Education and Awareness:** Educating family members, friends, and colleagues about the nature of cluster headaches, their impact on daily life, and available support resources can promote empathy and reduce stigma. Increased awareness fosters a supportive environment conducive to coping and adaptation.
- **Seeking Support:** Joining support groups, both online and in-person, provides individuals with cluster headaches and their caregivers with opportunities to connect with others

facing similar challenges, share coping strategies, and receive emotional support. Peer support networks offer validation, encouragement, and a sense of belonging.

4. Professional Support:

- **Counseling and Therapy:** Individual or family counseling can help individuals with cluster headaches and their loved ones navigate emotional challenges, improve communication skills, and develop coping strategies. Therapeutic interventions such as cognitive-behavioral therapy (CBT) can address maladaptive coping patterns and promote resilience.
- **Care Coordination:** Engaging with a multidisciplinary healthcare team, including neurologists, psychologists, social workers, and patient advocates, facilitates comprehensive care and support. Care coordination ensures that individuals with cluster headaches receive holistic management addressing physical, emotional, and social needs.

Conclusion: Cluster headaches have a profound impact on relationships and social functioning, affecting not only individuals with the condition but also their loved ones and caregivers. Understanding the challenges faced by individuals with cluster headaches in maintaining relationships and participating in social activities is essential for providing compassionate and comprehensive care. By fostering open communication, seeking support from peers and professionals, and implementing coping strategies, individuals with cluster headaches can navigate the challenges of living with this debilitating condition while maintaining meaningful connections and social engagement. Collaboration between healthcare providers, patients, and their support networks is crucial for addressing the multifaceted impact of cluster headaches on relationships and social functioning.

Coping Strategies and Support Systems

Living with cluster headaches presents numerous challenges, but effective coping strategies and robust support systems can help individuals manage symptoms, navigate daily life, and maintain overall well-being. This subchapter explores various coping strategies and support systems that individuals with cluster headaches can utilize to enhance their resilience, improve quality of life, and foster a sense of empowerment in the face of this chronic condition.

1. Coping Strategies:

- **Pain Management Techniques:** Employing pain management techniques such as relaxation exercises, deep breathing, guided imagery, and distraction techniques can help individuals cope with the intense pain associated with cluster headaches. These techniques can provide temporary relief and promote a sense of control over symptoms.
- **Stress Reduction:** Stress exacerbates cluster headache attacks for many individuals, making stress reduction techniques essential coping tools. Mindfulness meditation, yoga, tai chi, and progressive muscle relaxation are effective methods for reducing stress and promoting relaxation.
- **Healthy Lifestyle Habits:** Adopting a healthy lifestyle can contribute to overall well-being and potentially reduce the frequency and severity of cluster headaches. Regular exercise, adequate sleep, balanced nutrition, and avoiding triggers such as alcohol and tobacco can help manage symptoms and improve resilience.
- **Cognitive-Behavioral Strategies:** Cognitive-behavioral

strategies, such as cognitive restructuring, problem-solving, and goal setting, can help individuals develop adaptive coping mechanisms and challenge negative thought patterns associated with cluster headaches. Cognitive-behavioral therapy (CBT) with a qualified therapist may be beneficial for individuals struggling with psychological distress.
- **Pacing and Self-Care:** Learning to pace activities and prioritize self-care is crucial for managing energy levels and avoiding burnout. Breaking tasks into manageable steps, setting realistic goals, and practicing self-compassion can prevent exacerbation of symptoms and promote overall well-being.

2. Support Systems:

- **Family and Friends:** Building a support network of family members, friends, and loved ones who understand and empathize with the challenges of living with cluster headaches is invaluable. These individuals can provide emotional support, practical assistance, and companionship during difficult times.
- **Support Groups:** Joining support groups, either in-person or online, allows individuals with cluster headaches to connect with others who share similar experiences. Peer support provides validation, encouragement, and a sense of belonging, fostering resilience and coping skills.
- **Healthcare Providers:** Establishing a collaborative relationship with healthcare providers, including neurologists, headache specialists, primary care physicians, and mental health professionals, is essential for comprehensive cluster headache management. These providers can offer medical treatment, psychological support, and guidance on coping strategies.
- **Patient Advocacy Organizations:** Patient advocacy organizations dedicated to headache disorders provide

valuable resources, educational materials, and advocacy efforts for individuals with cluster headaches. These organizations offer information on treatment options, research developments, and access to community support networks.

3. Education and Empowerment:

- **Self-Education:** Educating oneself about cluster headaches, including triggers, symptoms, treatment options, and coping strategies, empowers individuals to actively participate in their care. Reliable sources of information, such as reputable websites, books, and medical journals, can help individuals make informed decisions about their health.
- **Advocacy and Awareness:** Advocating for oneself and raising awareness about cluster headaches can help reduce stigma, improve understanding, and promote access to appropriate care and support. Participating in advocacy efforts, sharing personal experiences, and educating others about the impact of cluster headaches can drive positive change.

Conclusion: Coping strategies and support systems are essential components of managing cluster headaches and promoting overall well-being. By implementing effective coping techniques, building strong support networks, and advocating for their needs, individuals with cluster headaches can enhance their resilience, improve symptom management, and maintain a sense of empowerment in their journey with this chronic condition. Collaboration between healthcare providers, support networks, and patient advocacy organizations is essential for providing comprehensive care and fostering a supportive environment for individuals living with cluster headaches.

Mental Health Interventions: Cognitive Behavioral Therapy, Counseling

Mental health interventions, including cognitive behavioral therapy (CBT) and counseling, play a crucial role in the management of cluster headaches by addressing the psychological impact of the condition and equipping individuals with effective coping strategies. This subchapter explores the principles and benefits of CBT, counseling, and other mental health interventions in the context of cluster headache management.

1. Cognitive Behavioral Therapy (CBT):

- **Principles:** CBT is a structured, evidence-based psychotherapy approach that focuses on identifying and modifying maladaptive thoughts, beliefs, and behaviors contributing to psychological distress. In the context of cluster headaches, CBT aims to help individuals develop adaptive coping strategies, challenge negative thought patterns, and enhance problem-solving skills.
- **Benefits:** CBT has been shown to be effective in reducing headache frequency, intensity, and disability, as well as improving mood, quality of life, and coping abilities in individuals with cluster headaches. By addressing psychological factors such as stress, anxiety, and depression, CBT can complement medical treatments and enhance overall well-being.
- **Techniques:** CBT techniques commonly used in the management of cluster headaches include cognitive restructuring, relaxation training, stress management, problem-solving skills training, and behavioral activation. These techniques help individuals develop more adaptive

responses to headache triggers, manage pain-related distress, and improve functional outcomes.

2. Counseling:

- **Role of Counseling:** Counseling provides a supportive and nonjudgmental environment for individuals with cluster headaches to explore their feelings, concerns, and coping strategies. Counseling sessions may focus on emotional processing, adjustment to the diagnosis, stress management, communication skills, and building resilience.
- **Types of Counseling:** Various types of counseling approaches may be beneficial for individuals with cluster headaches, including individual counseling, couples counseling, family therapy, and group therapy. The choice of counseling modality depends on individual needs, preferences, and available resources.
- **Integration with Medical Treatment:** Counseling can complement medical treatment by addressing psychological factors that may exacerbate cluster headache symptoms or impede treatment adherence. Collaborative care between healthcare providers and counselors ensures a holistic approach to cluster headache management.

3. Self-Help Strategies:

- **Psychoeducation:** Providing individuals with cluster headaches and their caregivers with accurate information about the condition, treatment options, and coping strategies is an essential aspect of self-help. Psychoeducation empowers individuals to actively participate in their care, make informed decisions, and advocate for their needs.
- **Self-Management Techniques:** Teaching self-

management techniques, such as relaxation exercises, stress management strategies, pain coping skills, and problem-solving techniques, empowers individuals to take an active role in managing their symptoms and improving their quality of life.
- **Peer Support Networks:** Engaging with peer support networks, such as online forums, support groups, and social media communities, provides individuals with cluster headaches with opportunities to connect with others facing similar challenges, share experiences, and exchange coping strategies. Peer support fosters a sense of belonging, validation, and encouragement.

4. Multidisciplinary Collaboration:

- **Integrated Care:** Collaboration between mental health professionals, neurologists, primary care providers, and other members of the healthcare team is essential for providing integrated and comprehensive care for individuals with cluster headaches. Coordinated care ensures that individuals receive holistic treatment addressing both physical and psychological aspects of the condition.
- **Treatment Planning:** Multidisciplinary treatment planning involves tailoring interventions to individual needs, preferences, and treatment goals. By considering the unique biopsychosocial factors contributing to each individual's experience of cluster headaches, healthcare providers can develop personalized treatment plans that optimize outcomes and improve quality of life.

Conclusion: Mental health interventions, including cognitive behavioral therapy (CBT), counseling, and self-help strategies, are integral components of comprehensive cluster headache management. By addressing psychological factors such as stress, anxiety, and depression, these interventions complement medical treatments and enhance overall well-being for individuals living with cluster headaches. Multidisciplinary collaboration between mental health professionals, neurologists, and other members of the healthcare team ensures holistic care and support for individuals with cluster headaches, empowering them to effectively manage their symptoms and improve their quality of life.

CHAPTER 8: FUTURE DIRECTIONS AND RESEARCH PERSPECTIVES

Novel Targets for Drug Development

Innovations in drug development for cluster headaches are crucial for addressing the unmet needs of individuals who do not respond to current treatments or experience significant side effects. This subchapter explores emerging targets and therapeutic approaches that hold promise for the future of cluster headache management.

1. Calcitonin Gene-Related Peptide (CGRP) Pathway:

- **Targeting CGRP Receptors:** CGRP is implicated in the pathophysiology of cluster headaches, with elevated levels observed during acute attacks. Monoclonal antibodies targeting CGRP receptors have shown efficacy in migraine prevention and are being investigated for their potential in cluster headache management.
- **CGRP Receptor Antagonists:** Small molecule CGRP receptor antagonists are also under development for

cluster headaches. These agents block CGRP signaling and may offer an alternative treatment option for individuals who do not respond to or tolerate other therapies.

2. Pituitary Adenylate Cyclase-Activating Polypeptide (PACAP) Pathway:

- **Role of PACAP:** PACAP is a neuropeptide involved in pain transmission and regulation of the trigeminovascular system. Preclinical studies suggest that PACAP signaling may contribute to cluster headache pathophysiology, making it a potential target for drug development.
- **PACAP Receptor Antagonists:** Selective antagonists targeting PACAP receptors are being investigated for their efficacy in cluster headache management. These agents may offer a novel approach to modulating trigeminal nociceptive pathways and reducing headache severity.

3. Serotonin (5-HT) Receptor Modulation:

- **Serotonin Receptor Subtypes:** Dysregulation of serotonin receptors, particularly 5-HT1B/1D receptors, is implicated in cluster headache pathogenesis. Novel compounds targeting specific serotonin receptor subtypes are under investigation for their potential in abortive and preventive treatment of cluster headaches.
- **Triptan Alternatives:** Triptans, which primarily target 5-HT1B/1D receptors, are effective abortive treatments for cluster headaches but may have limitations in terms of efficacy and tolerability. Developing alternative agents with improved pharmacokinetic profiles and receptor selectivity is a focus of ongoing research.

4. Neuroinflammation and Glutamate Modulation:

- **Role of Neuroinflammation:** Neuroinflammatory processes, including activation of glial cells and release

of pro-inflammatory cytokines, may contribute to cluster headache pathophysiology. Targeting neuroinflammation and glutamate signaling pathways represents a novel approach to preventing and treating cluster headaches.
- **Glutamate Receptor Antagonists:** Agents that modulate glutamate receptor activity, such as NMDA receptor antagonists or metabotropic glutamate receptor (mGluR) modulators, are being explored for their potential in cluster headache management. These compounds may attenuate excitotoxicity and reduce neuronal hyperexcitability associated with cluster headaches.

5. Non-Neuronal Targets and Immune Modulation:

- **Role of Mast Cells and Immune Cells:** Mast cell activation and immune system dysregulation may contribute to neuroinflammatory processes and trigeminal sensitization in cluster headaches. Targeting non-neuronal cells and immune mediators represents a novel therapeutic strategy for cluster headache management.
- **Immunomodulatory Agents:** Immune modulators, including monoclonal antibodies targeting inflammatory cytokines or immune cell receptors, are being investigated for their potential in cluster headache treatment. These agents may suppress neuroinflammation and mitigate the underlying immune dysregulation associated with cluster headaches.

Conclusion: Novel targets for drug development hold promise for advancing the treatment landscape of cluster headaches. Targeting pathways involved in trigeminal nociception, neuroinflammation, neurotransmitter modulation, and immune regulation offers new opportunities for developing more effective and tolerable therapies for individuals with cluster headaches. Continued research efforts aimed at elucidating the pathophysiological mechanisms of cluster headaches and identifying druggable targets are essential for advancing the field and improving outcomes for affected individuals.

Advancements in Neuromodulation and Neurostimulation

Neuromodulation and neurostimulation techniques offer promising avenues for the management of cluster headaches by modulating neural activity and disrupting pain pathways. This subchapter explores recent advancements in neuromodulation and neurostimulation technologies, including devices and techniques that have shown efficacy in the treatment of cluster headaches.

1. Occipital Nerve Stimulation (ONS):

- **Mechanism of Action:** Occipital nerve stimulation involves the implantation of electrodes near the occipital nerves, which are believed to play a role in the pathophysiology of cluster headaches. Electrical stimulation of these nerves modulates pain signals and may disrupt headache pathways.
- **Efficacy:** Clinical studies have demonstrated the efficacy of occipital nerve stimulation in reducing the frequency, intensity, and duration of cluster headache attacks, as well as improving quality of life. ONS is particularly beneficial for individuals who do not respond to or tolerate conventional treatments.
- **Implantable Devices:** Implantable neurostimulator devices, such as the Occipital Nerve Stimulator (ONS) system, deliver electrical pulses to the occipital nerves via implanted leads connected to a pulse generator. These devices can be programmed and adjusted to optimize treatment outcomes for individual patients.

2. Transcutaneous Vagus Nerve Stimulation (tVNS):

- **Stimulation of the Vagus Nerve:** Transcutaneous vagus nerve stimulation involves the non-invasive application of electrical stimulation to the auricular branch of the vagus nerve, typically via a handheld device placed on the outer ear. Stimulation of the vagus nerve modulates autonomic function and may exert anti-inflammatory and neuromodulatory effects.
- **Clinical Evidence:** Clinical trials evaluating the efficacy of transcutaneous vagus nerve stimulation for cluster headaches have shown promising results, with reductions in attack frequency, severity, and medication use reported. tVNS is well-tolerated and has a favorable safety profile.
- **Portable Devices:** Portable tVNS devices, such as gammaCore®, deliver targeted stimulation to the vagus nerve without the need for implantation. These devices offer convenience and flexibility for individuals with cluster headaches, allowing for on-demand or prophylactic use.

3. Deep Brain Stimulation (DBS):

- **Invasive Neuromodulation:** Deep brain stimulation involves the implantation of electrodes into specific brain regions implicated in pain processing, such as the hypothalamus or periaqueductal gray matter. Electrical stimulation of these regions modulates neural activity and may disrupt pain pathways.
- **Research Findings:** Preliminary studies investigating deep brain stimulation for cluster headaches have shown promising results, with reductions in attack frequency, intensity, and disability reported. DBS is considered a last-resort option for individuals with severe, refractory cluster headaches who have not responded to other treatments.

- **Surgical Procedure:** Deep brain stimulation requires a surgical procedure to implant the electrodes and pulse generator. Close collaboration between neurosurgeons, neurologists, and pain specialists is essential for patient selection, electrode placement, and postoperative management.

4. Supraorbital Nerve Stimulation (SNS):

- **Stimulation of Supraorbital Nerves:** Supraorbital nerve stimulation involves the placement of electrodes near the supraorbital nerves, which innervate the forehead and scalp. Electrical stimulation of these nerves modulates pain signals and may provide relief from cluster headaches.
- **Clinical Studies:** Clinical trials investigating supraorbital nerve stimulation for cluster headaches have shown promising results, with reductions in attack frequency, intensity, and medication use reported. SNS is well-tolerated and may offer an alternative or adjunctive treatment option for individuals with cluster headaches.
- **Implantable Devices:** Implantable neurostimulator devices for supraorbital nerve stimulation deliver electrical pulses to the targeted nerves via implanted leads connected to a pulse generator. These devices can be programmed and adjusted to optimize treatment outcomes for individual patients.

Conclusion: Advancements in neuromodulation and neurostimulation technologies hold promise for improving the management of cluster headaches. Techniques such as occipital nerve stimulation, transcutaneous vagus nerve stimulation, deep brain stimulation, and supraorbital nerve stimulation offer novel approaches to modulating pain pathways and reducing headache severity. Further research and clinical studies are needed to optimize these therapies, refine treatment protocols, and identify patient populations most likely to benefit from neuromodulation and neurostimulation interventions. Collaboration between healthcare providers, researchers, and industry partners is essential for advancing the field and improving outcomes for individuals with cluster headaches.

Precision Medicine and Personalized Therapies

Precision medicine and personalized therapies have emerged as promising approaches in the management of cluster headaches, aiming to tailor treatment strategies to the individual characteristics and needs of patients. This subchapter explores the principles and applications of precision medicine in cluster headache management, including the integration of genetic, biomarker, and clinical data to optimize treatment outcomes.

1. Genetic Profiling:

- **Genetic Variants:** Genetic factors play a role in the susceptibility to cluster headaches and response to treatment. Genome-wide association studies (GWAS) have identified genetic variants associated with cluster headache susceptibility, including variants in genes involved in circadian rhythm regulation, neurotransmitter signaling, and pain modulation.
- **Individualized Risk Assessment:** Genetic profiling allows for individualized risk assessment and stratification of patients based on genetic predisposition to cluster headaches. Identifying genetic markers associated with treatment response can guide the selection of personalized therapies and optimize outcomes.
- **Pharmacogenomics:** Pharmacogenomic approaches aim to predict drug response and optimize medication selection based on an individual's genetic profile. Genetic

variants affecting drug metabolism, receptor sensitivity, and drug transport can influence treatment efficacy and tolerability in cluster headache patients.

2. Biomarker Identification:

- **Biomarker Discovery:** Biomarkers are measurable indicators of disease activity, treatment response, or prognosis. Identification of biomarkers associated with cluster headaches, such as inflammatory markers, neuropeptides, and neuroimaging findings, can aid in diagnosis, monitoring disease progression, and predicting treatment response.
- **Predictive Biomarkers:** Predictive biomarkers help identify patients likely to respond to specific treatments and guide personalized therapy selection. Biomarker-based algorithms can inform treatment decisions, monitor treatment response, and adjust therapy accordingly to optimize outcomes.
- **Non-Invasive Monitoring:** Non-invasive biomarkers, such as serum biomarkers, neuroimaging markers, and digital health technologies, offer convenient and accessible means of monitoring disease activity and treatment response in cluster headache patients.

3. Clinical Phenotyping:

- **Patient Subgroups:** Cluster headaches exhibit heterogeneity in clinical presentation, symptomatology, and treatment response. Clinical phenotyping aims to categorize patients into distinct subgroups based on phenotypic characteristics, such as headache frequency, severity, duration, and associated symptoms.
- **Tailored Treatment Strategies:** Tailoring treatment strategies to specific patient phenotypes allows for personalized and targeted interventions. Phenotype-

driven approaches consider individual patient characteristics, comorbidities, treatment preferences, and lifestyle factors to optimize therapeutic outcomes and improve patient satisfaction.
- **Longitudinal Monitoring:** Longitudinal assessment of clinical phenotypes enables tracking of disease progression, treatment response, and treatment-related adverse events over time. Integrating longitudinal data with genetic and biomarker information provides a comprehensive understanding of disease trajectories and informs personalized treatment plans.

4. Multimodal Treatment Approaches:

- **Integrated Care:** Personalized therapies for cluster headaches often involve multimodal treatment approaches that combine pharmacological, non-pharmacological, and procedural interventions. Tailoring treatment regimens to individual patient needs and preferences maximizes treatment efficacy and minimizes adverse effects.
- **Shared Decision-Making:** Shared decision-making between patients and healthcare providers is essential for developing personalized treatment plans. Informed discussions about treatment options, potential benefits, risks, and patient preferences empower patients to actively participate in their care and make informed decisions.
- **Continuum of Care:** Personalized therapies for cluster headaches encompass a continuum of care that extends beyond acute symptom management to include preventive strategies, lifestyle modifications, and psychosocial support. Comprehensive care addresses the multidimensional needs of patients and promotes holistic well-being.

Conclusion: Precision medicine and personalized therapies offer a promising approach to optimizing the management of cluster headaches by tailoring treatment strategies to the individual characteristics and needs of patients. Integrating genetic profiling, biomarker identification, clinical phenotyping, and multimodal treatment approaches enables personalized decision-making and improves treatment outcomes. Continued research and innovation in precision medicine are essential for advancing the field and delivering more effective and individualized therapies for individuals with cluster headaches.

Printed in Dunstable, United Kingdom